BIPOLAR DISORDER(S)

How Controlling Light May Improve
Sleep and Reduce the Risk for
Episodes of Mania and Depression

RICHARD L. HANSLER PHD

© 2017 Richard L. Hansler PhD
All rights reserved.

ISBN: 1979036845
ISBN 13: 9781979036849

ACKNOWLEDGEMENTS

I want to thank my wife, Wanda Hansler, for her willingness to let me pursue my book-writing venture at an age when most men are retired. I also want to thank my children and grandchildren for their support and love. I also wish to acknowledge the support of my partners in Photonic Developments LLC, Dr. Edward Carome, Vilnis Kubulins, Dr. Martin Alpert, and Daniel Carome. I also owe a debt of gratitude to my granddaughter, Leah Hansler, and daughter, Susan Thomsen, who edited the manuscript and son-in-law, Mark Thomsen, who designed the cover.

PREFACE

Bipolar disorder is very likely a spectrum of disorders. Most varieties seem to be inherited in the form of mutations to some of the genes that make up the internal or circadian clock. Since genetic research is advancing very rapidly and to some extent is reaching clinical level, those with the disorder can expect rapid improvements in treatment options. There is a good case for doing genetic testing to validate treatment and to advance the testing itself. Establishing the physiology of the disorder(s) will help to dispel the stigma associated with bipolar disorder.

I, the author, am not a medical doctor, so nothing in this book should be regarded as medical advice. Hopefully, most suggested changes in behavior will be seen as common sense changes.

As a research physicist, I did research for GE Lighting for more than forty years, helping to make better and brighter light bulbs. After retiring from GE and moving to John Carroll University, I began studying the effect of artificial light on health. I learned that using light (especially blue light) in the hours before bedtime increased the risk for deadly illnesses. I feel guilty for my part in harming millions of people. In 2005, my partners and I opened a website where we sell products to allow people to avoid blue light. I am part owner of the company that operates the website, LowBlueLights.com. Our primary motivation continues to be to help people achieve better health.

If any of my readers want to know more about me, I did an interview with Tom Manos about my adventures during WWII. It is available on YouTube by searching Richard Hansler B17.

The US government maintains a database of abstracts (and in many cases, full papers) of medical studies conducted all over the world. The abstracts are searchable with a single number. Whenever an abstract is referenced in this book, its database number is cited in parentheses. I suggest you visit the database at www.pubmed.gov.

I hope that reading this book will increase your knowledge of bipolar disorder and add to your empathy for those struggling with this disorder. I hope it will help to dispel the stigma and discrimination associated with mental illness.

INDEX

Acknowledgements · iii

Preface · v

Chapter 1   What is Bipolar Disorder and
            How Does it Affect People? · · · · · · · · · · · · · · 1

Chapter 2   The Internal or Circadian Clock · · · · · · · · · · · · 17

Chapter 3   Genetic Aspects of Bipolar Disorder · · · · · · · · · 25

Chapter 4   How Environmental Factors
            Affect Bipolar Disorder · · · · · · · · · · · · · · · · · 49

Chapter 5   Is Bipolar Disorder Progressive? · · · · · · · · · · · 61

Chapter 6   Treating Bipolar Disorder · · · · · · · · · · · · · · · 71

Chapter 7   The Bottom Line · 91

CHAPTER 1

What is Bipolar Disorder and How Does it Affect People?

Definition

According to the National Institutes of Health:

Bipolar disorder, also known as manic-depressive illness, is a brain disorder that causes unusual shifts in mood, energy, activity levels, and the ability to carry out day-to-day tasks.

There are four basic types of bipolar disorder; all of them involve clear changes in mood, energy, and activity levels. These moods range from periods of extremely "up," elated, and energized behavior (known as manic episodes) to very sad, "down," or hopeless periods (known as depressive episodes). Less severe manic periods are known as hypomanic episodes.

Bipolar I Disorder— defined by manic episodes that last at least 7 days, or by manic symptoms that are so severe that the person needs immediate hospital care. Usually, depressive episodes occur as well, typically lasting at least 2 weeks. Episodes of depression with mixed features (having depression and manic symptoms at the same time) are also possible.

Bipolar II Disorder— defined by a pattern of depressive episodes and hypomanic episodes, but not the full-blown manic episodes described above.

Cyclothymic Disorder (also called cyclothymia)— defined by numerous periods of hypomanic symptoms as well numerous periods of depressive symptoms lasting for at least 2 years (1 year in children and adolescents). However, the symptoms do not meet the diagnostic requirements for a hypomanic episode and a depressive episode.

Other Specified and Unspecified Bipolar and Related Disorders— defined by bipolar disorder symptoms that do not match the three categories listed above.

Signs and Symptoms

People with bipolar disorder experience periods of unusually intense emotion, changes in sleep patterns and activity levels, and unusual behaviors. These 54distinct periods are called "mood episodes." Mood episodes are drastically different from the moods and behaviors that are typical for the person. Extreme changes in energy, activity, and sleep go along with mood episodes.

People having a manic episode may:	People having a depressive episode may:
• Feel very "up," "high," or elated • Have a lot of energy • Have increased activity levels • Feel "jumpy" or "wired" • Have trouble sleeping • Become more active than usual • Talk really fast about a lot of different things • Be agitated, irritable, or "touchy" • Feel like their thoughts are going very fast • Think they can do a lot of things at once • Do risky things, like spend a lot of money or have reckless sex	• Feel very sad, down, empty, or hopeless • Have very little energy • Have decreased activity levels • Have trouble sleeping, they may sleep too little or too much • Feel like they can't enjoy anything • Feel worried and empty • Have trouble concentrating • Forget things a lot • Eat too much or too little • Feel tired or "slowed down" • Think about death or suicide

Sometimes a mood episode includes symptoms of both manic and depressive symptoms. This is called an episode with mixed features. People experiencing an episode with mixed features may feel very sad, empty, or hopeless, while at the same time feeling extremely energized.

Bipolar disorder can be present even when mood swings are less extreme. For example, some people with bipolar disorder experience hypomania, a less severe form of mania. During a hypomanic episode, an individual may feel very good, be highly productive, and function well. The person may not feel that anything is wrong, but family and friends may recognize the mood swings and/or changes in activity levels as possible bipolar disorder. Without proper treatment, people with hypomania may develop severe mania **or depression.**

End of quotation from National Institutes of Health

Incidence

Dr. James Phelps, psychiatrist and author of "Bipolar Spectrum Disorders", believes that bipolar disorder is not a single disorder but a range of similar disorders including schizophrenia. He maintains a very valuable website www.psycheducation.org.

A number of famous people are believed to have suffered from bipolar disorder. Vincent Van Gogh is regarded as the "poster person" for Mental Health month. Winston Churchill was never diagnosed but showed symptoms of bipolar disorder. Many high-profile successful people, including Robert Kennedy Jr., Kim Novak, Demi Lovato, Catherine Zeta-Jones and Jean-Claude Van Damme have been diagnosed with bipolar disorder, once known as manic depression.

The incidence of bipolar disease in the US is estimated at 2.7% of the population, or 5.7 million people. An estimated 60 million people suffer from bipolar disorder globally. If you know 37 people, one of them may be suffering from bipolar disorder. The damaging effects of the disorder become clearer when reading people's own accounts of what it is like to have a bipolar disorder. A selection of these accounts is provided below. For a better understanding of how bipolar disorder affects lives, the author also recommends that readers search for the many excellent videos on this topic on YouTube.

Personal Accounts
"My Bipolar Disorder And I Aren't Friends, But We're Getting Along Better Now"

Posted by Bijoy Jose in Mental Health

May 24, 2017

I used to think of mental illness as taboo for a very long time until my personal experience with it. Now, I've grown to accept mental illness as just another way for the body to communicate its priorities. I'm sharing my experience with Bipolar Disorder hoping it can resonate with others who have had mental health difficulties at some point in life. I think an important message that I take away from it is that I am not alone – love unites us.

Toughest Phase of My Life- First Episode and being diagnosed as Bipolar

I was diagnosed with Bipolar Disorder in 2012. At the age of 26 – it was one of the toughest phases of my life. It started with a period where I experienced episodes of high anxiety, worry and fear which I also believe was triggered due to certain situational factors, followed by episodes of Mania.

Mania Phase – The High Phase

Mania for me can be described as moments where I considered myself supreme without a weakness. I started judging and thinking less of others around me. Something I think I've always chosen to stay away from earlier. This phase can be categorized as a stage with a very high ego – something I now choose to live without and the blurring between what is real and not (unrealistic feelings like someone wants to hurt me). The tough part about Mania is the inability to know that something is wrong. It had gotten really terrible at one point that the lack of sleep and insufficient rest over a period of days had got me hallucinating at which point my sister noticed the difference in my behavior.

Family and Friend's Support – A critical factor to identify a mental illness

My sister has been a great support. She recognized a difference both in my behavioral traits and a marked difference in my manner of acting and offered to take me to a psychiatrist. When she told me, I resisted and was in denial – I didn't want to visit the doctor. I kept thinking that I was absolutely well. In hindsight, I was not in a position to understand what I was going through. This was followed by episodes of sudden change in my emotions – yet there I was in a stage of mania where I felt I was being a very big person by going with my sister to meet the doctor. I feel blessed to have a caring family and a wonderful friend who supported me through that period.

Tackling the Denial Phase- Meeting the Psychiatrist

Before meeting the doctor I felt a sense of immense fear that I don't totally understand. However as mentioned having my sister and cousins come with me and be my side enabled me to meet with the psychiatrist. He initially prescribed medication that put me to sleep for a period of close to two days where I just woke up, had my meals and went back to sleep. I still remember how the medicines helped me get out of the period of Mania and I was beginning to feel a bit normal (before mania phase) again.

Guilt Phase – What was I thinking?

Things were slowly beginning to feel better for me personally; however, the tough phase was not over yet. This period epitomizes my intense guilt I had for feeling the way I did during my mania phase, mostly for thinking I was faultless and supreme. I wondered why I had these thoughts, this illness and a feeling of worthlessness.

Depression Phase

In continuum came the period where I began to feel I was worthless and alone – this again is a phase where I undervalued myself and began to feel that I am no good. This again is an unreal phase since I was unable to identify my strengths and primarily looked only at my weaknesses and my negative thoughts were all I had. It was also a phase, in which I was unable to be productive with an incredible amount of my time. This again was the scariest period since I had thoughts of suicide that slid by without my knowledge. The cycle of Mania and Depression so far has been the toughest period for me.

Acceptance Phase – Importance of Medication and Identifying Triggers

Apart from the medicines which play an important role in managing the illness – another critical part is to know the triggers to of Mania and Depression with Bipolar illness:

Sleep: I've observed that sleep is important for me to function at my best. I make it a point to at least sleep for a period of eight to ten hours which is what my body requires at the moment.

Intoxicating substances: I've realized the need to keep a check on alcohol consumption for me and the need for avoiding any other substance that alters my behavior.

Medication: I am on Lithium & Quitipin and have been for the past four years. I hope there comes a time when I don't need medication – but that is something I would have to rely on my doctor's opinion on whom I trust

Self-Control: Another aspect of the illness is to act less on impulses. I am making an effort to be conscious of my impulses and then either delay or take steps to not indulge them.

Stop Fearing and Continue Loving: I believe that anger, worry, and anxiety are certain things that affect our mental health a great deal. Essentially, I've come to believe that loving each other and also importantly forgiving oneself and others constantly are key to a more healthy and happy living.

Self-Awareness, a key to better mental health:

Mental illness is tough since it is of the mind and you're fighting yourself. Beyond the medicines, self-awareness is a constant pursuit. Most important to better mental health, is the love you receive and share to all. I do think that illnesses of the mind are also communicating something very important – it helped me better understand my actions and my thoughts; feelings and emotions. I've begun to believe that challenges are only a way to get to know your inner self better. Am I going to face more challenges, maybe yes but I choose resilience always!

Experiences shared are personal and intended for the intent of breaking the taboo around mental illness and society's acceptance, empathy towards those experiencing it.

Bijoy Jose is a social entrepreneur – a postgraduate (MSW) from Tata Institute of Social Sciences, Mum

"Bipolar Musings: On Mania & Being Muslim"

by Karen Kaiser

July 4, 2017

I always hear that suicide is haram and that someone who dies by suicide will be forever punished for this act. In fact, I've been lectured about this on numerous occasions. This statement of fact is where the discussion usually ends; in my experience, anyway.

And though I can recall lectures, khutbahs, and khatirahs explaining why suicide is forbidden, I've not heard any discussion on how to avoid this as a Muslim living with mental illness. For someone like me, who has a mind that constantly sees suicide as a way out of pain & misery, the lack of advice in this area is detrimental to my health. I'm still looking for practical tips to help me avoid this grave deed.

I've had to seek outside assistance for real world advice on healing from suicidal thoughts and ideation. In fact, I've learned the most valuable lessons on how to access my Iman and strengthen my connection with Allah during suicidal moments from religious people of other faiths. Over the years I've come to realize that refusal to address an issue that's uncomfortable or frightening doesn't make it go away. And it doesn't erase the fact that people struggle with it in their daily lives.

Getting tattoos is haram in Islam as well. However, this is something I'm inclined to do during periods of mania. Indulging in any vice, really. Everything haram or shameful suddenly seems amazing when I'm manic. Nothing is unattainable in those moments. And everything seems like the best idea you've ever had. Mania is a saboteur in that way.

What is Bipolar Disorder and How Does it Affect People?

Someone once asked why I got tattoos when I was manic. I was defensive at first because I couldn't rationally explain why I'd do something I knew to be haram. Later, I realized a simple fact. "This is mania!" This is exactly how it works. Mania knows no religion, and certainly is not inclined to respect specific religious edicts and rules. Mania has no moral compass, no understanding of boundaries. Mania is that terrible yet seductive friend, whose only job is to be an enthusiastic cheerleader for all things exciting, dangerous and risky.

Thinking about my experiences with mania, I remembered back to a conversation I'd had years ago with an intake nurse from a nationally acclaimed health organization. The nurse was asking me questions about symptoms I experienced during manic episodes, to qualify me for an important medical study. "During a typical episode: Do you stop sleeping, and for how long? Do you stop eating? Do you dress differently, more provocatively? Do you spend excessive amounts of money or engage in impulse buying? Do you over indulge in drugs/alcohol? Have you gotten tattoos/piercings? Do you engage in risky relationships or dangerous situations?" I couldn't listen anymore. The humiliation of embarrassing things I'd done during euphoric manic periods was overwhelming. I panicked. I abruptly cut the nurse off and interjected, "ok I'm a practicing Muslim, ma'am. Some of those questions don't apply to me. I'm not supposed to do things like that."

She paused. Then gently said, "bipolar disorder (or any mental illness) doesn't care what religion you are. Anyone can become ill and experience the symptoms associated with a condition, despite what they believe in. If you're saying you haven't done these things, then you haven't had a true manic episode. I'd further suggest that the diagnosis of bipolar I disorder is inappropriate for you. And in that case, you're ineligible for this study."

That's not what I'd intended at all. I just couldn't face my mistakes in that moment. But missing out on cutting edge treatment simply because I was embarrassed at how mania had impacted my life seemed ill advised. I corrected myself. "Ok. I understand what you're saying. That makes sense", I softly admitted. She asked if I'd like to continue the intake process. "Yes." I whispered. She resumed her questions, and this time I answered honestly.

I've learned that what happens when I'm manic is a direct result of my mental illness and not something that has to do with character, morals or manners. It's the definition of what it means to live with a mental illness, and nothing more. I no longer stigmatize myself as to the mistakes I make during mania, because I realize that I'm doing the best I can within my limitations. That's all I can ask of myself.

"Never give up on finding the right medicine"

By Hattie Gladwell

Friday 16 Jun 2017

Throughout my school years, my weight fluctuated. I'd always been a little bit chubby and it was something that I was self-conscious about. It had a massive impact on my self-esteem.

But by the time I reached the age of seventeen, I'd managed to lose the weight and my confidence sky-rocketed. I felt the best I'd ever felt. I didn't realize what confidence was until I finally felt okay in my body.

A few years later, I found myself becoming the insecure girl I'd so desperately wanted to leave in the past.

At the age of twenty I was diagnosed with bipolar disorder after having episodes of both mania and depression, and severe, uncontrollable outbursts. Immediately, I started medications prescribed by a psychiatrist, including quetiapine, a form of anti-psychotic.

The medication was wonderful. I went from an erratic, quick-to-tempered girl to a calm and collected woman.

While I had episodes of mania and depression still, they were controlled with the meds. For the first time in a long while, I felt as though my head was clear. I was able to process things and walk away from negative situations as opposed to rising to them and making things worse.

But over time, while my head felt less out of control, my self-esteem was plummeting.

The medication was making me gain weight – which, unfortunately, is a common side effect with quetiapine. Of course, it affects everyone differently, but for me, it made me gain a stone over just a couple of months.

My weight was a big thing for me – it's something that can easily get me down, and, having found confidence in my body since being a size I liked, the pros and cons of the medication were at a tie.

I knew that if I kept gaining the weight, my self-esteem would get dramatically worse, and would start affecting my mental health more so than the medication.

And so, I asked my psychiatrist to stop the medication, and he trialed me on something new. The next medications were Respiridone and Abilify – two other forms anti-psychotic.

They were awful. They made me feel constantly sick. My weight didn't shift and I suffered with headaches and disorientation.

Again, I went back, and asked to change.

This time, my psychiatrist asked me the pros and cons of each medication I'd been on so far and what I wanted from each medication.

I told him I wanted to be stable, I wanted to be functional, and I didn't want it affecting my weight. As many mental health medications affect your weight, the list of medications available to me became short. But I didn't lose hope.

I was prescribed Lithium – a mood stabilizer. Alongside this, I was given Chlorpromazine, another anti-psychotic.

The chlorpromazine was a god-send. It allowed me to think clearly, my temper decreased, and all in all they made me feel happy within myself.

The Lithium helped keep my episodes stable – if I had a manic episode it lasted for a shorter amount of time than they previously had, and I didn't do anything too impulsive while taking it.

But over the course of taking it, I found that my weight was changing, again. While it wasn't as dramatic as previous medications, I gained a stone over the course of six months – four pounds of which were gained while I was on a carb-free diet. Alongside the (smaller) weight gain came the inability to lose it. It didn't matter what I did or what I ate, the weight refused to shift.

I was often very dehydrated – which is another side effect of Lithium. Being dehydrated affected my sleep and gave me headaches.

The medication also caused me to sweat a lot, no matter what I wore.

I developed acne – which left me feeling insecure without makeup, especially as even through my teenage years, I only ever had to deal with the occasional spot.

And so back to the psychiatrist's office I went.

What is Bipolar Disorder and How Does it Affect People?

And I'm glad I did. I'd trialed enough medications now to speak with him honestly about my side effects and how they were affecting my mental health, and finally he suggested putting me on a medication that he'd been hesitant to do so beforehand. Lamotragine.

Lamotragine is a type of mood stabilizer that is often not prescribed straight away as it can be very addictive. If the dose isn't heightened in a slow manner then the side effects can be dangerous – including a nasty rash that can be lethal.

I was just willing to try anything else to get me by, and I wanted to give it a go.

I have been trying out Lamotragine for six weeks now. It started with the smallest dose and has since gone up to a standard one, as I wait another four weeks to go up to the full dose. Over this time, I've been kept on Lithium to ensure that while the Lamatrogine gets into my body, I still have a mood-stabilizer being absorbed.

Because of the Lithium, I can't really say how well things are working, but what I have found is that since being on the Lamotrogine, it has been easier to lose weight. My skin has cleared up a little and there have been no negative side effects besides the occasional nausea.

I really think this is the medication that I've been waiting for over the past two years, and I'm so glad I'm finally finding one that works for me.

My story isn't just to talk about taking medication, though. It's to talk about why it's important not to give up on it.

When you're suffering with a mental illness it can be really hard to see any light at the end of the tunnel. And it's frustrating when seeking help to struggle to find something that works for you.

It's easy to think it'd be better to just give up and go medication-free – even though that's often not a safe option.

It's so important to stick out all of the trial and errors instead of losing hope.

Put it this way: if you were trying to get fit, you wouldn't try one type of exercise, then give up on your health entirely when you find that exercise doesn't suit you, would you?

No, you'd do a circuit around the gym trying to find something that is going to get you where you want to be.

And that's exactly the way you've got to look at it in terms of mental health medication. It's all trial and error. It's tiring, it's time consuming, and you likely will experience some side effects along the way. But always remember your main goal: to get better.

Never lose that focus, because if you keep going, eventually you will find something that works for you – and you'll look back and feel so glad that you never, ever gave up on bettering your mental health.

Chapter 1 Summary

Bipolar disorder is a complex spectrum of disorders, and everyone with bipolar disorder has a different story. The treatment must therefore match the individual.

The reader will learn in Chapter 2 that certain characteristics of light, especially the time of exposure and the color, disrupt the body's circadian rhythm. This disruption can exacerbate the damaging symptoms of bipolar disorder. Thus, there is promising evidence that light-related interventions may be universally beneficial to people who suffer from bipolar disorder.

CHAPTER 2

The Internal or Circadian Clock

Author's Note: A huge body of research exists on the circadian clock; according to pubmed.org, more than 13,000 technical papers have been published on the topic. Readers are encouraged to refer to PubMed for more information and/or to view the papers cited in this chapter.

Understanding the Circadian Clock

In order to understand how light affects people with bipolar disorder, we need to learn about the internal or circadian clock. Almost all living things have some means for keeping track of time, which allows them to predict and prepare for the future. It's fun to think of all the ways nature has programmed living organisms to work on a schedule, including seasonal as well as daily schedules.

Perhaps the most striking are the many animals that change their colors. Mammals may change the color of their fur: brown in summer, white in winter. Birds often develop brilliant colors or build nests to attract a mate at the right time of year. Many animals become fertile in the fall or winter, so the young are born in the spring, when the chance of survival is highest. Many birds, animals and even butterflies migrate with the changing seasons. All these activities must be done at the right time.

The Internal or Circadian Clock

On a shorter time-scale, the organs in living organisms adjust their activities throughout the 24-hour day. The term "circadian" means literally "about a day". For example, the liver needs to produce bile in connection with when food is consumed. A corned beef sandwich eaten at 11PM may not go down as well as one eaten at noon. The kidneys slow down production of urine at night, which prevents us from waking up every couple of hours. The organs and individual cells throughout the body all have local clocks.

The local clocks are synchronized by the master clock that is located in the hypothalamus at the base of the brain, in what is called the suprachiasmatic nucleus (SCN). The master clock follows a cyclical 24 hour schedule as follows: The master clock is synchronized with the rotation of the earth and is reset every morning when the eyes are exposed to natural daylight, especially blue light. Approximately 12 hours later (in the early evening), the clock sends a signal to the pineal gland to start producing melatonin. This informs melatonin receptors, located in organs and tissues, that it is nighttime, time to rest and renew. The concentration of melatonin in the blood stream gradually increases to a maximum about six hours later, during sleep, and then drops to near zero, about wake up time. This circadian cycle then repeats itself.

When humans first evolved, we lived near the equator where there are 12 hours of light and 12 hours of darkness year-round. The re-setting of the clock occurred when the sun came up. When darkness came, melatonin began flowing. This all worked well until people moved away from the equator. Now the clock also needed to be a calendar and predict the changing seasons.

About a century ago, experiments were done in which people moved into caves or other places where there were no means for telling what time it was. Their so-called "free running" clocks continued to keep them on a daily pattern but with days slightly longer than 24 hours, about 24.4 hours. This is referred to as "Non 24". Blind people experience this same situation. They do not experience the daily resetting of their clock because their eyes are not exposed to light in the early morning. This means they may have melatonin present during the day when they want to be awake, and experience poor sleep at night. It was discovered in the 1990s that taking a small amount of melatonin at the same time every day would keep the internal clock synchronized with the earth's rotation. Vanda, a pharmaceutical company, has developed and patented a drug very similar to melatonin that also will reset the internal clock if taken at the same time every day. Interestingly, they advertise their product by showing its benefits for a blind person.

Genes controlling the master clock

Throughout nature there are internal clocks of many different degrees of sophistication. They are put together in modular fashion, where different modules are added to improve function when adjusting to different circumstances, such as the changing light duration when moving away from the equator. The change in the duration of darkness becomes the calendar.

The things that are doing the equivalent of "ticking" in a mechanical clock are genes and proteins produced from the genes. In the simplest biological clock, a portion of the DNA is "opened" for copying by a promoter gene called "Clock". It is copied by genes called "Per" and "Cry", and a protein is produced which is then gradually eliminated in a chemical process. Each of these steps requires a certain length of time. The clock is restarted when the eyes are exposed to light in the morning, which sends a signal to the SCN that activates a gene called Rev-erb to restart the process. In humans, the clock is much more complex, as is illustrated in the following figure:

Figure 1. Illustration of Master Circadian Clock in Humans

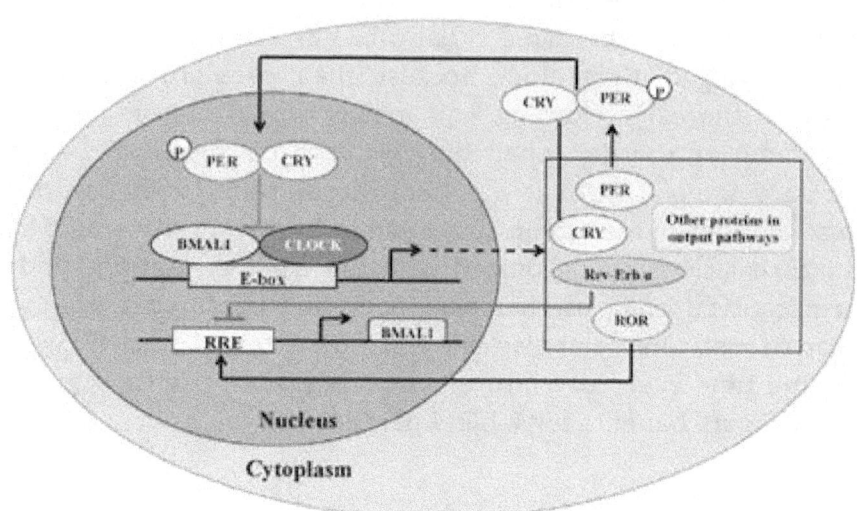

It is important to understand the operation of the internal or circadian clock because bipolar disease is at least partially the result of gene mutations, some of which are the genes making up the internal clock.

How the circadian clock relates to Bipolar Disease

There is increasing evidence that at least some people with bipolar disorder are affected by the duration of daylight. Typically these individuals experience an increased risk of developing mania in the spring as the hours of daylight are increasing. Some psychiatrists talk about "May mania". Following is a discussion of several scientific studies documenting the relationship between the circadian clock and psychiatric disorders.

A 2017 study (27988807; see Preface for meaning of this number) found that there was no difference in the expression of the major clock genes under dim or bright light except for REV-erb beta that is involved in the morning resetting of the clock. It was more strongly expressed by bright light.

Another 2017 study (28468274) describes in part the relationship between clock genes, altered sleep-wake rhythms and psychiatric disorders as follows:

> "Circadian clocks enable organisms to anticipate temporal organization of biological functions in relation to periodic changes of the environment, and to adapt consequently their behavior. The genes Clock, Per, Cry and Bmal1 are currently the major clock genes identified in humans as being involved in the rhythmicity and timing of biological rhythms at the molecular level. Their alteration involves changes to the 24-h rhythm through poor synchronization between the endogenous circadian rhythms and the sleep-wake cycle, and act especially on sleep disorders. These are often early symptoms of altered sleep–wake rhythms at the onset of psychiatric disorders, especially for mood disorders. Furthermore, impairments in the four major clock genes (Clock, Per, Cry and Bmal1) were found for bipolar disorder, depression-related disorders, autism spectrum disorder, and impairments in some of these major clock genes were also reported for schizophrenia (Clock, Per and Cry), anxiety disorder (Cry) and attention deficit hyperactivity disorder (Clock). In addition, other clock genes were associated with these psychiatric disorders, such as Npas2 (winter depression, autism spectrum disorder and schizophrenia), RORA and RORB (bipolar disorder) or Tim, Dbp and Ck1ε (autism spectrum disorder). The associations of identical clock genes with these different psychiatric disorders suggest that they may share similar pathways and etiopathogenic mechanisms. It highlights the interest and need to study these mental disorders through a transnosographic and multidimensional approach focusing on depression, anxiety and stress responses."

Another 2017 study (28264500) examines the overlap of genes associated with autism, bipolar disorder and schizophrenia. It concludes:

> "The convergence of pathways governing circadian rhythms supports the existence of a common core etiological relationship between neuropsychiatric illness and sleep disruption possibly related to central brain stem dysfunction impacting the presentation and underlying pathology and course of illness."

The relationship between the circadian clock and bipolar disorder is established in a 2016 study (27543154) whose title contains the results of the study, **"Advanced Circadian Phase in Mania and Delayed Phase in Mixed Mania and Depression, Returned to Normal after Treatment of Bipolar Disorder."** "Advanced circadian phase" means the clock is set to an earlier hour than normal, which creates effects like the flow of melatonin starting sooner in the day than normal.

If the genes making up the circadian clock are defective as a result of genetic mutations, the disruption of the circadian rhythm may result in poor sleep and psychiatric problems. A second source for disruption of the circadian rhythm can be exposing the eyes to artificial light at night (ALAN) in the hours before bedtime or during the night, as in shift work.

A 2016 study (27308960) is titled **"Circadian Disruption: New Clinical perspective of disease pathology and basis for chronotherapeutic intervention."** It documents the results of the disruption as follows:

> "A surprisingly large number of medical conditions involve [circadian disruption]: adrenal insufficiency; nocturia; sleep-time non-dipping and rising blood pressure 24 h patterns (nocturnal hypertension); delayed sleep phase syndrome, non-24 h sleep/wake disorder; recurrent hypersomnia; SW intolerance; delirium;

peptic ulcer disease; kidney failure; depression; mania; bipolar disorder; Parkinson's disease; Smith-Magenis syndrome; fatal familial insomnia syndrome; autism spectrum disorder; asthma; byssinosis; cancers; hand, foot and mouth disease; post-operative state; and ICU outcome."

If the clock genes contain mutations and the clock does not provide the correct time, it can also affect the metabolism. A 2015 paper (26483181) is titled **"Circadian Clocks as Modulators of Metabolic Comorbidity in Psychiatric Disorders"**. It documents how obesity and diabetes may arise from dis-regulation of glucocorticoid, dopamine, and orexin/melamine concentrating hormone systems.

A 2015 study (26317159) is titled **"Mice lacking circadian clock components display different mood-related behaviors and do not respond to chronic lithium treatment."**

Actually, the study included mice expressing Per2, Cry1, and Rev-erb alpha that did respond to lithium treatment, suggesting their significant role in the circadian clock and in bipolar disorder. Mice missing the Cry1 gene displayed the co-existence of both manic and depressive symptoms.

A large 2015 study (26283580) compared the genomes of 473 Latino family members with bipolar disorder with the genomes of 411 family members free of bipolar disorder. They identified mutations in two circadian genes that appear to be associated with bipolar disorder. Several other circadian genes may be associated with bipolar disorder.

There is not universal agreement that mutations in the genes of the circadian clock are associated with bipolar disorder. A 2014 study (24687905) found none of the gene mutations of clock genes were associated with bipolar disorder, schizophrenia or major depressive disorder.

There are a number of people who are referred to as experiencing Delayed Sleep Phase Disorder and live as "Night Owls". They typically go to bed at 3 AM and sleep until 11AM or later." This makes it difficult to live a normal life. Whether this is a problem with the circadian clock is not clear. In any event it appears it is difficult for them to change their lifestyle.

An interesting sidelight to this discussion is a 2014 study (25358694) titled **"Genetic adaptation of the human circadian clock to day-length latitude variations and relevance for affective disorders".** The author suggests the circadian clocks of humans 200,000 years ago in Africa did not include the ability to deal with change in day length. When humans migrated away from the equator where day length varies, evolutionary changes that provided the increased capability of the clock to accommodate changes in day length may have also resulted in the mutations that produced bipolar disease and other affective disorders.

Chapter 2 Summary

Whether bipolar disorder is caused by mutations in the genes that comprise the circadian clock still remains to be proven, though the scientific literature seems to point toward this conclusion. There is strong evidence that some of the symptoms of bipolar disorder (e.g. poor sleep) involve the circadian clock. In the next chapter, we will look at the relationship between genetics and bipolar disorder.

CHAPTER 3

Genetic Aspects of Bipolar Disorder

Bipolar disorder is a disorder that is found in families, generation after generation. As mentioned in the last chapter, the mutations of genes that make up the circadian clock appear to be associated with bipolar disorder. Other genes may also be associated with bipolar disorder. At present, we are in the midst of rapidly expanding studies of the genetics of mental diseases. Because of this rapid expansion of knowledge, anything you read here may very quickly be out of date. We will examine what is currently known and how this knowledge may be helpful to those with this disorder.

Studies of Bipolar Disease in the Amish Community

The studies of bipolar disorder in the Old Order Amish of Lancaster County, Pennsylvania have contributed much to our still limited knowledge of the genetics of bipolar disorder.

1. The abstract of a 1988 paper (3164866) is included here to provide background:

Pharmacopsychiatry. 1988 Mar; 21(2):74-5. **A genetic study of manic-depressive disorder among the old order Amish of Pennsylvania.**

Egeland JA1

Genetic Aspects of Bipolar Disorder

Abstract

"A genetic and epidemiological study of the genetic linkage of major affective disorders is being conducted for over 10 years among the Old Order Amish in Pennsylvania, a genetic isolate leading a uniform pattern of life. An autosomal dominant mode of inheritance was found to be most consistent with the transmission patterns in the Amish families. The advent of DNA technology suddenly revolutionized the field of genetic linkage studies. The finding that major affective disorders were linked to DNA markers on the short arm of chromosome 11 was reported in "Nature" as a first report of the location of a dominant gene conferring a strong predisposition to a common psychiatric condition. A strong linkage was shown to two DNA markers, insulin and the cellular oncogene Haras-1. Several other candidate genes should also be studied, for example, the structural gene encoding for tyrosine hydroxylase (TH gene). It is important to ask why certain people "at risk" remain well, whereas others develop major affective disorders. An effort is also underway to test whether other forms of affective disorder are part of the same genetic spectrum. The Amish study has to maintain a research strategy of interface between psychiatry and other scientific disciplines."

Autosomal dominant is one of several ways that a trait or disorder can be passed down (inherited) through families. In an autosomal dominant disease, if you inherit the abnormal gene from only one parent, you can get the disease. Often, one of the parents may also have the disease.

II. The human side of the story of bipolar disorder in the old order Amish community can be seen in this account of the doctors treating these families for the past 40 years:

"The link between genetics and mental illness continues to engage Abram Hostetter, a psychiatrist in his fourth decade of world-recognized research into why Old Order Amish are more susceptible to bipolar disorder than the general population.

Hostetter, an alumnus of two Mennonite colleges, is part of a University of Miami team that has been researching mental illness among generations of Amish families in Lancaster County since 1976.

He and project leader Janice Egeland, professor of psychiatry, behavioral sciences, epidemiology and public health at the University of Miami, worked for years together out of an office in Hershey, Pa. They assembled a team of about a dozen others to assist them.

"The Old Order Amish of Lancaster County have a lower incidence of mental illness than the general population, but a much higher incidence of bipolar disorder," Hostetter said.

Bipolar disorder, also called manic depression, sometimes leads to suicide.

"It's in the blood," said an Amish grandmother — or *siss im blut*, in Pennsylvania German — when Egeland began her research.

Bipolar disorder is characterized by episodes of mania or depression that typically recur and often become more frequent and severe during a lifetime. It is estimated that about 1 percent of the U.S. population has a major mood disorder.

Over the years, scientists discovered an association between mood disorders and two known genetic markers. In other words, people suffering from bipolar disorder have inherited it from their parents.

Hostetter and Egeland found that Old Order Amish families are ideal subjects for genetic studies for a number of reasons:

- They descend from a limited number of pioneer couples who came to America in the 18th century.

- There is little marriage to outsiders or other forms of in-migration, causing the Old Order Amish of Lancaster to form a closed gene pool.

- They have large families and keep extensive genealogical records.

- They prohibit the use and abuse of alcohol and drugs, which often mask the symptoms of bipolar disorder.

"We have a total pedigree of the Old Order Amish community in a computer from the original 32 adults who came in the 1760s until in the 1970s," Hostetter said, "so we can determine what percentage of genetic endowment any two people share."

The research team focuses on the original "pedigrees," or cohort. About 65 percent of the families are named Stoltzfus. Other names are King, Zook, Lapp, Beiler, Petersheim, Blank, Fisher, Miller, Glick, Esch and Smoker.

Hostetter grew up in Lancaster County and knew some Amish families with bipolar disorder. His grandfather, a longtime moderator of Lancaster Mennonite Conference, often consulted with Amish ministers. Hostetter's father was a farmer and tobacco broker and also had much interaction with the Amish.

"My best friend, an Amish boy, in elementary school had bipolar disorder, as did his mother and grandmother," Hostetter said. "He committed suicide at age 18, and his sister committed suicide in the 1990s."

Hostetter was a pre-med major at Eastern Mennonite University in Harrisonburg, Va., for two years in the late 1940s. He earned his bachelor's degree from Goshen (Ind.) College in 1953. He graduated from Jefferson Medical College in Philadelphia and trained in psychiatry at Norristown State Hospital.

He joined a private practice in his home area and later formed a group practice in Hershey, where he met Egeland, who was on the faculty of Hershey Medical Center.

"We first spoke about using the Amish population in Lancaster County to solve the medical puzzle about inheritance of bipolar disorder in 1970," he said.

Egeland and Hostetter both joined the faculty of the University of Miami but worked out of what they called "University of Miami, North Office" in Hershey.

Nine years ago Hostetter retired from his psychiatry practice at age 74 and moved with his wife to Charlottesville, Va. He returns to Pennsylvania about five times a year, though, to pursue his research. In December, he joined Egeland there.

"We worked on 'coding' cases to detect particular characteristics of each of their manifestations of illness," he said. "We have very detailed medical histories and DNA samples on over 100 bipolar patients.

At this point we are on the verge of whole genome sequencing for 80 subjects, still attempting to locate all the specific genes involved."

Bipolar disorder is treatable, and people with the illness can lead normal lives.

"However, untreated or inadequately treated, there is still a 15 percent suicide rate, to say nothing of the suffering and turmoil these people have and put their families through," he said."

END OF QUOTATION.

III. The full genome for 388 Amish family members was studied and the results published in a 2014 paper (24625924). The conclusion from the abstract is as follows:

"However, despite the in-depth genomic characterization of this unique, large and multigenerational pedigree from a genetic isolate, there was no convergence of evidence implicating a particular set of risk loci or common pathways. The striking haplotype and locus heterogeneity we observed has profound implications for the design of studies of bipolar and other related disorders."

There is no one "smoking gun" but a number of clusters of genes, some or all of which are associated with the bipolar disorder experienced in this isolated community.

IV. More useful information is contained in this account of a program involving Amish children:

Why the Amish Are a "Living Laboratory" For Research in Bipolar Disorder

In many ways the Amish community provides a natural laboratory for all genetic and clinical and phenomenological research. It is a well-defined, closed population with little migration into or out of the community. The community can trace its ancestry back to 30 progenitors in Switzerland, and it maintains extensive genealogic records. The Amish community encourages a high birth rate, so a researcher can study large families. It is also important that this community prohibits the use of alcohol and drugs—substances known to complicate prenatal health as well as diagnostic ascertainment and assessment.

Finally, while the Amish have no more bipolar disorder than any other population group, they have always viewed bipolar disorder as a medical condition ("Siss im blut"—it's in the blood, as they say), and they seek medical care for what they view as medical illnesses.

Dr. Egeland has been conducting genetic and epidemiological studies among the Old Order Amish since 1976 and has had a long-standing, trusting relationship with this community. Her earlier studies have identified families with a high loading of bipolar I disorder under genetic linkage study, and she can now look at the fourth and fifth generation of children as she has known many of their parents since the parents were babies themselves.

The Study Design and the Hypothesis

The Child and Adolescent Research Evaluation (CARE) program of the Amish study was initiated in 1994 and was designed to follow a group of 210 children and adolescents in two samples: a bipolar I sample and a control sample. The bipolar I sample were the children of a parent who was known to have bipolar I disorder. The control sample consisted of children who had a well parent whose sibling had the disorder, and a group of children with a family history negative for any psychiatric illness.

The hypothesis of the study was that there would be a gradation of risk for bipolar disorder: with children of one parent with the illness having the highest risk, followed by children whose parents were well but had a sibling diagnosed with the disorder (nieces and nephews), and by children in families with no history of the illness having the lowest rating of risk.

If this hypothesis were correct, the goal would be not only to gauge the genetic risk factors, but to identify the temperamental features and behaviors that might be predictors of an eventual manifestation of the illness.

At the time of recruitment in 1994, 14 candidate bipolar I families (8 fathers and 6 mothers with the illness) were invited and agreed to participate. A matched control group was assembled with children of same-sex psychiatrically-unaffected parents who had a sibling with the illness. Because it was not possible to obtain a sibling control for all the families, the parent with bipolar disorder was matched by sex, age, and family size to an unrelated Amish man or woman with a family history that was negative for psychiatric illness.

The final sample of 210 children consisted of 100 children from 14 families where a mother or father had bipolar I disorder; 77 children from 9 control families where the parents had a sibling who had bipolar disorder; and 33 children from four control families with a history negative for the illness.

How Was the Information About the Children Collected?

In order to launch the study that would follow children and adolescents over a twelve- to fifteen-year period, Dr. Egeland and her colleagues and a group of child psychiatrists, child development scientists, a pediatrician, and Amish advisors developed a formal schedule of questions that became known as the CARE Interview. This interview covered medical and developmental histories (Part A), a health narrative (Part B), and a third questionnaire with 69 inquiries related to a wide range of symptoms and life events (Part C). Part C's questions were considered comprehensive enough to reveal potential early or prodromal features of bipolar illness.

The parents were asked whether their child was "noticeably different" from "other boys and girls" his or her own age. In the Amish community there are such well-defined roles for children, with specific chores expected at various ages that role performance (and any possible impairment) can be detected quickly.

Amish children have no homework after school. They go right home, go upstairs and change their clothes and go out and do their chores. Therefore, if these chores are completed in an inconsistent or spotty fashion, the parents realize that something is wrong. This is important because "role impairment" (functioning) is an element in psychiatric assessment. Hence, parental rating of chores gives a measure of "wellness" for each child annually.

How the Children Were Evaluated for Possible Risk

After a mother answered Part A of the CARE Interview, both parents answered Parts B and C, and the narrative file for each child was presented randomly to the CARE panel. This panel was composed of two board-certified child psychiatrists, a board-certified general psychiatrist, and a clinical psychologist.

All members of the panel were totally blind to the children's identity or family history.

The panel members independently coded CARE narratives in sets of 10 children and recorded their clinical opinion for risk of developing a bipolar disorder. The options the doctors had to code these well children included high risk, moderate risk, low risk (these codes indicated the highest risk ratings); well with a BP tag; or well with no evidence of risk.

The "BP tagged" risk category was used for children who were well, but who were manifesting some clinical features that suggested a possible onset of bipolar disorder in years to come, but who did not at this time warrant a risk rating. Risk rating represented a "clinical judgment" based on the substantial clinical experience of the panel, and there had to be consensus about each rating.

Which Group of Symptoms Occurred Most Frequently in Which Group of Children?

When all the data were assembled and the statistical analyses performed, the children of a bipolar parent were reported to have manifested more clinical features on the coding sheet than the control group, and the children of well parents who were siblings of a bipolar I patient manifested more clinical features than the children with no family history of psychiatric illness.

To add in the statistics: When rated for risk, 38% of the bipolar sample (compared to only 17% of the control sample) had high-moderate-low -ratings. Yet the vast majority of children in the control sample who had risk ratings, turned out to be the children who had an aunt or uncle with the illness (83%).

Similar to other studies of genetic risk, the children at highest risk had a parent with the illness. Children with a second-degree relative had a reduced risk but this risk was still higher than the risk for those who came from families negative for any psychiatric disorder.

Because we don't want anyone to misinterpret the statistics, it is important to point out that the 38% figure is not the genetic risk factor to a child of a parent with bipolar. These Amish children are well with certain symptoms/features, and—depending on how many of the children onset with the illness—these symptoms/features may be suggestive of an early symptom profile for bipolar disorder.

The genetic risk to a child of one parent who has the illness is usually pegged between 20 and 30%. However, no one knows which factors may forestall an illness from developing and which genes might even be protective.

Which Clinical Features or Symptoms/Behaviors Did the At-risk Children Have?

The children who had a parent with bipolar I disorder had a statistically significant higher frequency for 10 clinical features when compared to the control group. Listed alphabetically they are:

- Anxious/worried
- Attention poor/distractible in school
- Energy low
- Excited
- Hyper-alert
- Mood changes/labile
- School role impairment
- Sensitivity
- Somatic complaints
- Stubborn/determined

It is interesting that the temperamental features of sensitivity, hyper-alertness, being anxious/worried or nervous appeared to be continuous as the parents responded to these with remarks such as "always" or "by nature." However, half or more of the reports about decreased or increased energy and mood were episodic and all but one report on anger/temper showed as periodic rather than continuous.

This differs dramatically from the ultra-ultra rapid-cycling pattern of mood, energy, irritability and temper problems reported in so many non-Amish children, and raises questions about environmental influences on the presentation of symptoms and course of illness.

The Temperamental Features of Being Hyper-alert Or Overly Sensitive

Seventy percent of the children at risk for bipolar disorder had parental reports mentioning how "hyper-alert" and "overly sensitive" the children were. In the retrospective study that Dr. Egeland reported on two years ago, one quarter of the adults with bipolar I disorder had hospital records that noted "overly sensitive compared to others" prior to onset. (That figure may have been higher, but these were chart reviews of first hospitalizations and the symptom profile was not probed systematically upon admission.)

Parents and teachers in the Amish community who identify a child as "overly sensitive" refer to a child who has a heightened sense of awareness. If one observes such children, their "social skin" appears to be overexposed. They may seem "hyper-alert" to the feelings of others—peers and adults alike. It is as though an electrical field surrounds these youngsters and their antennae pick up all possible signals.

According to Dr. Egeland, "They seem to notice everything: how someone is dressed, whether their shoes are shined…they get very close to you and seem to need some physical contact. If another child gets stung by a bee, this child will feel so deeply that she will cry for the injured child."

It has long been known that people in a manic state are hyper-alert, hyper-vigilant, and hyper-sensitive. According to the authors of the Amish findings, these features of being "overly sensitive" and "hyper-alert" could be early predictors of bipolarity.

Dr. Egeland then mentioned something that struck us when she added: "These children feel things very intensely and they are oversensitive to color."

Parents who participated in the original survey for The Bipolar Child also mentioned this overall sensitivity; and one area of particular sensitivity was to color. One mother described her young daughter as "very sensitive in the visual realm. She is drawn like a magnet to some designs and colors, beautiful paintings, landscapes, and repelled by others, as strongly as she reacts to odors and tastes."

When one looks at the art of Peter Paul Rubens, Vincent Van Gogh, Maurice Utrillo, Edvard Munch, and Jackson Pollack (all of whom suffered with manic-depression) it is easy to see this important sensitivity to color.

The Symptoms and Cycling Patterns Of The At-Risk Amish Children In Contrast To Non-Amish Children

More severe symptoms and symptoms of mania tend to manifest later in Amish children—most likely in adolescence. In this population, symptoms were showing up in the prepubertal years, going underground, and reemerging in adolescence. Also of interest, the Amish children of a bipolar I parent were not at a higher risk for patterns of disruptive behaviors, oppositional behaviors, or the hyperactivity so often seen in prepubertal children diagnosed with the disorder in communities outside the Amish culture. The authors write:

It is interesting that in our prospective study, clinical features such as mood, increased and decreased energy, decreased sleep, and anger/temper were noted to occur periodically in 50% or more of the reports for children of a bipolar parent. Other studies have suggested that the most frequent pattern of prodromal symptoms of bipolar disorder is characterized by continuous and chronic manifestations of irritability, mood dysregulation, and rapid cycling with little inter-episode relief.

What accounts for these differences in presentation is not known, but it is interesting to speculate whether the absence of alcoholism within the Amish community may differentially influence the presentation of the illness in comparison with non-Amish families.

What Next?

According to Dr. Egeland and the other authors of this article, the research in the CARE study now rests on the ultimate outcome of a bipolar disorder diagnosis for a well child correctly designated "at risk." The researchers plan to follow the children for 12 to 15 years and will be reporting new findings in the literature throughout that period of time. A new article is expected sometime next spring.

In the meantime, genetic markers in one or more chromosomal regions for susceptibility gene(s) have been established in adults with bipolar disorder in the Amish community, and the researchers are collecting DNA from a number of the children in the CARE program. As this program is the only prospective study with the goal of comparing clinical prediction and genetic patterns for bipolar disorder, future reports from the Amish study will no doubt do much to expand our knowledge of the genetics, the early symptoms, and the course of childhood-onset bipolar disorder.

In Conclusion

Amish children live in a completely pacifistic society where anger or violence are never displayed, and where they are expected to be well-behaved, submissive to authority, quiet and non-intrusive around adults. Their opinions are never asked for or expressed. These children have never seen television, the nightly news or scary or gory movies, and they have never played Nintendo. They use no electricity and tend to go to sleep soon after nightfall and arise early with the sun—their sleep patterns are extremely uniform. They also have many brothers and sisters who act as role models, and are surrounded by cousins and peers who follow the traditions of the community closely and thus provide an additional abundance of role models. The social structure that surrounds children in this community is practically impossible to duplicate.

And yet, Amish children who have early symptoms of a possibly evolving illness cannot always conform to the expectations of their culture—anymore than can children suffering with these symptoms in the world outside."

Janice Papolos and Demitri Papolos, M.D.

END OF QUOTATION.

V. Another benefit of the genetic studies of the Amish is explained in this article by Edward I, Ginnis published in Mar. 11, 2015 issue of Psychology Today:*

Genetic Aspects of Bipolar Disorder

Do you know what Abraham Lincoln, Vincent Van Gogh, Ernest Hemingway and Marilyn Monroe have in common? If you guessed they all had bipolar disorder, you're right.

Recently we identified a key genetic pathway underlying bipolar disorder that may lead to new, more effective drugs to treat it and other mood disorders, such as depression.

The roots of our discovery started in the 1960s, when Janice Egeland, currently professor emerita at Miami's Miller School of Medicine, began studying the health practices of Old Order Amish families of Pennsylvania. She found that a rare form of dwarfism—called Ellis-van Creveld syndrome—and bipolar disorder were prevalent among an extended family traced back to one individual. Indeed, the rate of bipolar disorder was extremely high.

But here is the surprise: No one in this family afflicted with the Amish genetic dwarfism had bipolar disorder. This suggested that the DNA change causing this dwarfism in the Amish was protective of bipolar disorder.

This dwarfism in the Amish results from DNA changes that disrupt a signaling pathway known as sonic hedgehog. This pathway—a series of chemical reactions—plays a key role in embryonic development, but it had never been connected to bipolar disorder.

Our research in the 1990s provided the first evidence for genes protective of bipolar disorder. This research, coupled with our recent surprising finding, supported the idea that the DNA change causing the pathway disruption in Amish dwarfism blocks bipolar symptoms.

If we can mimic this positive protective effect, we can create new drugs to more effectively treat the disease. Also, there are drugs currently studied that target the chemical reactions in the sonic hedgehog pathway for other medical conditions. These same drugs may be beneficial in the treatment of bipolar disorder in adults.

We still have a lot of work to do before we fully understand bipolar disorder. The sonic hedgehog pathway involves more than a dozen molecules and interacts with many other genes. It is likely that changes in other genes or proteins in this pathway may be involved in determining the course of the disease.

I feel privileged to pursue this research with many talented colleagues, and I hope others will be inspired to do so, too. Highly effective treatment for bipolar disorder and other mental illnesses can be a reality.

END OF QUOTATION.

The abstract of the technical paper about the previous study may be found by searching PubMed for 25311364.

Because of the complexity of the genetic basis for bipolar disorder, various ways to focus the search are being developed. One such study (245222887) from 2014 looked at isolated communities in the central valley of Costa Rica and Antioquia. The study included 738 individuals, of which 181 have bipolar disorder one (BP1). The characteristics (phenotypes) that are both heritable and associated with BP1 were found to be the cortical thickness in the prefrontal and temporal regions of the brain, and the volume and micro-structural integrity of the corpus collosum. Genetic studies have not yet been published, but this means of narrowing the search seems promising.

Bipolar Parents

Some bipolar parents have regrets they were not diagnosed before they had children. Here are their stories:

Stacey Galka, 38, of Denver, is a single mom who was diagnosed with bipolar disorder when she was 26. At that point, her daughter was already 5 years old. Stacey says her own diagnosis was a relief because it helped her to make sense of why her life had always been so chaotic, but when her daughter was diagnosed with bipolar disorder at age 13, Stacey had trouble accepting it. "In all honesty, if I had known then what I know now, I would have never had a kid," she says. "It was difficult enough for me to go through what I did."

While the chances of some children having bipolar disorder are heightened by genetic factors, there are ways of treating the illness. Ronald R. Fieve, MD, a psychopharmacologist in private practice in New York City, notes that medications have revolutionized the lives of people living with bipolar disorder and provided successful treatments.

In order to mitigate the onset of bipolar disorder in any at-risk child, however, Dr. Fieve says that general health is very important: normal sleep patterns, a healthy diet, regular exercise, and the avoidance of drugs and alcohol. Sleep deprivation or major life stresses can precipitate the onset of a manic or depressive episode.

Brandi, 34, lives in Colorado Springs. She was diagnosed after her first pregnancy kicked her into a manic episode, and medications have stabilized her moods. Now, she has two daughters. Although she worries that they'll inherit the disorder, she says she is more concerned about how her own bipolar disorder may affect her. As a bipolar parent, she tends to yell and make bad decisions with food or shopping, and gets easily agitated when her symptoms flare. "I do worry that they're going to end up with something. I keep a close eye on my 3-year-old," she says. "I have to keep telling myself, 'This is normal 3-year-old behavior. She's just fine. So I guess it's not a matter of being afraid of her being bipolar so much as I'm afraid of how she's going to turn out because of *my* bipolar."

Genetic Testing for the Diagnosis of Bipolar Disease

The field of bipolar diagnosis is experiencing progress, as illustrated by the following articles:

I. A genetic test for bipolar?

"Genetic Testing and Depression, Anxiety and Bipolar Disorder: Could a Simple Cheek Swab be the Missing Link in Your Mental Health Treatment?

What is Genetic Testing Targeted to Mental Health and How Does it Help?"

Written by Dr. Bruce Kehr

We have all heard about the rise in at-home, direct-to-consumer genetic testing by companies such as 23andMe. But what you haven't been hearing much about from your psychiatrist is genetic testing targeted to your specific mental or emotional health issue. This is called Pharmacogenomics, originally developed by the Mayo Clinic and Cincinnati Children's Hospital in 2013 with Assurex Health. Identifying certain genetic markers, called pharmacogenetic markers, in a patient can shed light on whether particular psychiatric drugs will be effective and whether there is a higher risk of adverse events from those drugs for that individual. Psychiatrists can tailor their treatment plan to each patient based on his or her pharmacogenetic markers, which include genetic mutations that predict alterations in how the underlying neurons and synapses (brain cells and their connections) function, and the rate that a patient metabolizes medications, to help avoid issues such as lack of effectiveness, drug-resistance and drug interactions. It's a more objective, evidence-based guidance system to help doctors select the right medication for their patients.

Our practice works with a company called Genomind, which is a leader in this type of precision medicine that focuses on treating the individual rather than a population. They developed a genetic test called the Genecept Assay® that uses a patented algorithm based on hundreds of studies to interpret a patient's test results, which doctors use to help decide the most appropriate class and dose of medication for each patient. In a recent study, clinicians reported that 87 percent of their patients showed improvement with treatment guided by the Genecept Assay®. They also reported improvement in 91 percent of patients who had failed at least two medications in the past. In February of this year, the federal government made veterans and active military personnel eligible to receive the Genecept Assay® as part of their treatment plan. The government capitalized on this technology in 2014 when Medicare and the U.S. Department of Veterans Affairs approved Assurex Health's test called GeneSight™. This is a trend that is only growing.

Is there Enough Evidence That Genetic Testing Guides Psychiatric Treatment Effectively?

Like any breakthrough, genetic testing in psychiatry is not without its controversy. The Boston Globe published an article in October of 2015 on the reliability of these new tests, focusing on an investigation conducted by the New England Center for Investigative Reporting (NECIR). NECIR examined studies conducted to determine the efficacy of genetic testing in treating depression and anxiety, and called into question the validity of results, because in many cases the studies were funded by the very companies that administer the genetic tests. This poses a potential conflict of interest that can't be ignored. Scientists have called for more large population-based studies to gather a larger pool of data, first to have an independent evaluation of genetic testing as a tool to treat mental illness, and second to help clinicians measure individual testing results against more established findings. Dr. Robert Klitzman, professor of psychiatry and director of the Bioethics Masters and Online Certificate and Course Programs at Columbia University, reminds doctors using genetic testing in their practice that life circumstances, and interpersonal and environmental interactions can shape many mental health conditions, not just a patient's genetic traits. It is important to understand that genetic testing is one of many possible interventions that guide diagnosis and treatment of psychiatric conditions; other lifestyle choices, such as your diet and any other medications you are taking, contribute to the effectiveness of antidepressants, antipsychotics and other psychiatric drugs. This is why a psychiatrist must still take a thorough history and use traditional clinical diagnostics in combination with genetic testing to evaluate and treat each patient.

Despite the criticism that genetic testing in psychiatry needs more regulation and research, psychiatrists do have access to published guidelines for use of pharmacogenetic testing and their effectiveness. Further, the Food and Drug Administration (FDA) has started to recommend genetic testing for specific psychiatric drugs and even include model for evaluating these tests based on analytical validity, clinical validity, clinical use, and the ethical information about pharmacogenetics on drug labels. An organization called the International Society of Psychiatric Genetics is one of many that monitors the ethical implications of this treatment intervention.

Genetic Testing is the Future of Mental Health

In January of this year, the New York Times reported that researchers for the first time can trace the onset of schizophrenia to a person's genetics. Scientists from Harvard Medical School,

Boston Children's Hospital and the Broad Institute found that a variant in a particular gene affects a process during adolescence where the brain sheds weak or redundant neural connections as the individual matures. Those who have overactive forms of the gene shed those neurons too quickly are more prone to schizophrenia. Although this finding is not enough to test the general population, testing for this gene in young people who already show early signs of the disorder could direct the course of their treatment in a potentially life-altering way. This is just the beginning of a revolution in psychiatric medicine. We are going to see breakthroughs that will shatter the status quo. Stephen M. Stahl, MD, PhD, Professor of Psychiatry University of California, San Diego (UCSD) said, "Psychiatrists and mental health professionals have long practiced personalized medicine, individualizing complex combinations of treatment for their patients. We are now on the brink of a new era where genomics such as through the Genecept Assay® can be added to the tools they use to select treatment options with the best chance of tolerability and efficacy." In a video that Dr. Stahl posted as part of the American Psychiatric Association 168th Annual Meeting in 2015, he says that psychiatrists should embrace genetic testing and be early adopters, because a person's genome will never change, but the science behind how we interpret a person's genome will only become more advanced.

Every practitioner should be aware of this technology and offer it as a treatment option to his or her patients. If your doctor has not recommended it to you or your loved ones yet, you should take the initiative and ask about it. You don't want to waste precious time living in a limbo where you are stable but not really getting better, when the answer could be just a cheek swab away.

END OF QUOTATION

II. "Genetic Testing Offers Hope to People with Bipolar Conditions"
By the Honorable Patrick J. Kennedy

After a 16-year career in Congress, today I'm dedicated to improving the lives of people around the world who are experiencing mental illness, addiction, and other brain diseases.

This means it is incumbent upon me to hear and learn from people with mental health conditions, including those dealing with bipolar conditions and depression.

One patient dealing with depression I know about is James Crawford

Let me share some of his story in the first person, as he has many times in the past:

As long as I can remember, I had been depressed. For me, depression was an exhausting fight against drowning.

Twenty years ago, when I was 24, my psychiatrist prescribed antidepressants, and I continued trying different ones for nearly two decades. It didn't seem to matter which ones I took, or how many, the affect was minimal, at best.

During this time I was also going to appointments for traditional talk therapy; it helped some, but, ultimately, it was like a donut filled with air; it just didn't feel substantial.

Finally, two years ago, a relatively new psychiatrist of mine suggested I take a genetic test to help guide my treatment. The goal was to look at the genes that may affect my body's ability to benefit from certain drugs and other treatments.

This testing finally offers some personalized, objective, biological markers that clinicians can use to understand what mechanisms may be going wrong in the brain to cause mental health conditions, and how to potentially correct them with drugs and other treatments. We have come to expect personalized medicine in many other areas of healthcare, such as in cancer, and now it is finally available for mental health as well.

The standard of care in psychiatry is and has been a trial-and-error process of prescribing drugs to lessen the symptoms of mental illness. It consists of trying one type of drug after another, and adjusting drug dosing until, hopefully, the patient feels better. This process can and often does take months or years, and many times the patient never reaches remission from his or her symptoms. Patients often lose hope and do not comply with their treatments. Sometimes, the drug side effects are so severe that patients totally abandon their regimen.

Genetic testing may serve to help reduce the stigma around mental illness, since it is an objective test that can assist in showing what may be physically going wrong to cause the condition. Hopefully this can help to further our effort to place mental health conditions in the same category as all other physical illnesses.

I'm happy to report that James recently got engaged. His story is one of thousands that show the potential that genetic testing holds as part of a successful treatment plan.

END OF QUOTATION.

CHAPTER 4

How Environmental Factors Affect Bipolar Disorder

The fact that bipolar disorder occurs in multiple generations in families establishes that there is a genetic basis. The second fact, that the symptoms do not appear at birth and may not occur until well into adulthood, establishes that environmental factors play a significant role. We will examine some of these environmental factors. The most compelling research examines how environmental factors play a role in controlling and stabilizing the circadian clock.

Circadian disruption

As mentioned in Chapter 2, mutations in some of the clock genes may result in circadian disruption in some people with bipolar disorder. Circadian disruption also occurs in millions of ordinary people due to exposure to ordinary electric lighting, and to some extent by sunlight for those who dwell far from the equator.

Since disruption of the circadian rhythm is known to be detrimental to living things, it is important to go into the details of how the circadian rhythm may be stabilized.

I. Light exposure and the circadian clock

The circadian clock is reset by exposure to light. It wasn't until 2001 that it was established that blue light (peak at about 460nm) is most effective in resetting the clock. Exposing the eyes to natural daylight (which is typically 10-10,000 times as strong as artificial light) is a great way to start the day. This process, called entrainment, keeps the circadian clock synchronized with the rotation of the earth.

During dark winter mornings, a brightly lit bathroom or kitchen can do the job. Light boxes specially designed for this purpose, are available. I suggest that investing in a bright ceiling fixture for the kitchen is a better investment than a light box. In addition, "dawn simulation lamps" are available that brighten gradually and wake you gently. Nice, but probably not necessary.

Human circadian clocks are quite stable. If you miss exposing your eyes to light one morning, your clock will still keep running and melatonin will begin flowing at the usual time in the evening, unless your eyes are exposed to light at that time.

A major function of the circadian clock is the control of the pineal gland that produces melatonin and a few other hormones. When melatonin travels throughout the body, it synchronizes the local (peripheral) clocks found in every cell. Melatonin also acts on the organs that control core body temperature. This results in a minimum body temperature about 18 hours following the re-setting of the clock in the morning, i.e. midnight.

If the eyes are exposed to bright light before this minimum body temperature, the clock will be set to a later hour. If exposed after the minimum, the clock will be set to an earlier hour. The stability of the master clock limits the shift to an hour or two. This is why you can't get over five hours of jet lag in one night.

In summary, the **blue component of light** is most important in controlling and resetting the circadian clock.

II. Peripheral clock setting

As with most controls in the body, there is a back-up system. The master clock in the suprachiasmatic nucleus (SCN) also sends out nerve messages that help to synchronize the peripheral clocks. In addition, there are other both external and internal stimuli that help to maintain the circadian rhythm.

Recent studies verify that eating at a regular time helps stabilize the circadian rhythm. There is evidence that the food entrainment of the clock includes a region of the brain different from the SCN's master clock. If you have ever been at a zoo at feeding time you know the animals are very aware it's time to eat. Our pet goat lets us know if it's past time to feed him.

a. Feeding Time

A 2015 study (26012377) is titled "**Feeding Time**" and describes (in not too technical language) how food can influence the internal time keeping.

> "All forms of life have to be able to cope with changes in their environment, including daily cycles in temperature and light levels. As a result, organisms as diverse as bacteria and humans have evolved inbuilt timekeeping mechanisms that are capable of tracking the 24-hour day.
>
> These so-called 'circadian' clocks enable organisms to anticipate changes that take place in their environment, and adapt their biology accordingly. In addition to tracking time, biological clocks must stay synchronized (or entrained) with the world around them. To achieve this, circadian clocks can be influenced or reset by environmental factors called 'zeitgebers' (from the German for 'time-giver'). The daily cycle of light and dark is a dominant

zeitgeber for most organisms, while periodic food availability represents another powerful zeitgeber. Now, in *eLife*, Henrik Oster and colleagues—including Dominic Landgraf and Anthony Tsang as joint first authors—report how a hormone released from the gut after eating can help the body to track changes in mealtimes (Landgraf et al., 2015).

Circadian clocks have a profound impact on mammalian biology, and virtually all aspects of our lives—from sleep-wake cycles to patterns of hormone release and energy metabolism—follow pronounced daily rhythms (Albrecht, 2012). In mammals, it is well established that the suprachiasmatic nucleus (or SCN) contains the body's master clock. Located in the brain, just above the optic nerves, the SCN clock receives information about environmental light levels directly from the eyes, which keeps it in sync with the external world.

Twenty years of research into circadian clockwork mean that we understand relatively well how changes in light adjust the timing of the SCN clock. The expression of specific 'clock genes', such as *Per1* and *Per2*, within neurons of the SCN are increased in response to light. This means that the SCN clock can be advanced or delayed to ensure it remains in time with the prevailing light–dark cycle. However, it has also become clear that there are other circadian clocks in most of the cells and tissues in the body (Guilding and Piggins, 2007; Mohawk et al., 2012).

Under normal circumstances, this network of clocks is kept in synchrony by the master clock in the SCN; but it has been known for many decades that behavioral rhythms in laboratory rodents can be entrained by restricting access to food to certain times of the day. These food-entrained rhythms are not affected by the light–dark cycle, and they can persist in animals that have had their SCN destroyed. A set mealtime is now known to be a dominant zeitgeber for these peripheral tissue clocks (such as the clock in the liver), with the expression of the clock genes in these tissues become aligned to feeding time (Damiola et al., 2000). In contrast, the SCN clock remains locked to the light–dark cycle. It makes sense for tissue-specific clocks to be sensitive to food instead of light because the availability of food in nature may not always coincide with other environmental factors.

Unlike modulation of the SCN clock by light, it is unclear which signals convey information about feeding time to reset the circadian clock in the liver. Oster, Landgraf, Tsang and colleagues—who are based at the Max Planck Institute for Biophysical Chemistry, and the Universities of Lübeck and Toronto—report that a gut hormone called oxyntomodulin is one of these signals. Oxyntomodulin is a peptide hormone that is released from the gut in response to food intake, and has been suggested to be a potential drug target to combat obesity in humans (Druce and Bloom, 2006).

Landgraf, Tsang et al. started by screening around 200 peptide molecules that are known to be involved in appetite and the regulation of body weight to see if any could adjust the molecular clock of liver tissue. This in vitro screen identified two molecules: oxyntomodulin and glucagon. In particular, treatment with oxyntomodulin could shift the liver clock by several hours, either forward or back, depending on the time it was administered. Both of these characteristics suggest that oxyntomodulin serves to set the liver clock to feeding rhythms in living organisms."

End of: "Feeding Time" article

b. Odor resetting

A 2015 study (233825589) is titled **"Odor is a time cue for circadian behavior"**.

In experiments with rats they found providing an odor at a certain time interval controlled the timing of behavior, e.g. use of running wheel. This was true in rats without an SCN as well as normal rats. This suggests that clocks in some peripheral cells are responsible.

c. Networks

Another 2015 study (26252253) is titled **"Synchronization of the mammalian circadian system: Light can control peripheral clocks independently of the SCN clock: alternative routes of entrainment optimize the alignment of the body's circadian clock network with external time."**

They describe a "federated" network of peripheral cells in various parts of the body that respond to timing of light exposure independent of the master clock in the SCN.

> "A "federated" network, however, allows for each clock and, therefore, each physiological process to be synchronized to those zeitgeber signals that are most relevant for a particular process, resulting in a tailored response. For example, the liver clock should be synchronized to rhythms in food intake, but it should also respond to changes in energy demands or variations in oxygen supply. A "federated" organization allows for better adaptation to changing environments. For example, seasonal adaptation of circadian rhythms might be facilitated by differential resetting of tissue clocks in response to changes in photoperiod, temperature, humidity, and other parameters that change over the course of a year."

III. Avoiding circadian disruption

Before electric lighting, when we used candles, kerosene lamps, and gas lights, there was little blue light in the flames. Even the early electric lights with carbon filaments produced a yellow light, not rich in the blue rays that affect the special sensors in the eye that control the circadian clock. Only the more modern light sources, like LEDs, are rich in blue light.

Evening exposure to modern lights and electronic screens disrupts our circadian rhythms. This disruption can easily be avoided by the use of light bulbs that don't make blue light. Or alternatively, one can wear orange glasses that block blue light. Wearing these glasses for several hours before bedtime can prevent any disruption of your circadian rhythm.

IV. Using circadian rhythm to treat bipolar disorder

As previously discussed, individuals with mutations in the genes that make up the circadian clock may develop bipolar disorder. If some components in your master circadian clock do not function normally, it may be possible to control your circadian rhythm through environmental factors. ***By keeping a regular schedule of waking, showering, eating, working, exercising, relaxing, and going to sleep, you can help overcome any deficiency in your "clock genes". In other words, regaining control of the circadian clock may help to relieve episodes of bipolar disorder.***

You can do the following to avoid the disruption of your circadian rhythm caused by evening exposure to light, especially blue light. As discussed earlier, if you expose your eyes to light at 7 AM, your body will start making melatonin at 7 PM, but only if blue light is avoided in the evening. Putting on glasses that block blue light or using light bulbs that don't make blue light will work. This will help to stabilize your mood and result in your body making as much melatonin as possible. It will also improve your sleep, which is a serious problem for many people with bipolar disorder.

Two studies in 2014 (24460899) and 2016 (26804589) describe why maximizing melatonin by controlling evening light is so effective. They describe the evidence that the pineal gland inserts melatonin directly into the brain by way of a passage into the third ventricle (hollow space) inside the brain. Melatonin is also introduced into the blood stream, but is in a higher concentration in the cerebrospinal fluid that bathes the brain.

The concentration of melatonin in the brain is important to people with bipolar disorder because some episodes of mania and of depression result in detrimental changes in the brain. Melatonin protects the brain from damage in many ways. For example, melatonin has been shown to neutralize reactive oxygen species produced by the very active brain during mania.

V. Other causes and effects of circadian disruption

a. City life

A Scientific American 2016 article is titled, "Does City Life Pose a Risk to Mental Health?" This article discusses research showing that growing up in the city doubles the risk of mental illness compared to the population as a whole. Some blame the 24/7 lifestyle that disrupts the circadian rhythm.

b. Daylight saving time

The twice yearly shift to and from daylight saving time is known to upset some people with mood disorders. Following is an article from PsychCentral:

> **"How will a longer stretch of dark mornings and light evenings affect us?"**

Written by Jane Collingwood

For one thing, we are all likely to become more active in the evenings.

Feeling that the best part of the day's not over when we leave work can't help but make us feel more optimistic, and outdoor exercise suddenly will be a nicer prospect! Social activities also are likely to increase when we're able to savor more daylight. An hour of light after work means more opportunity for ball games, trips to amusement parks and shopping.

Other benefits may include a drop in crime, as people are not out so much in the dark, and an estimated drop in road traffic injuries, as people are leaving work and school in daylight. However, traffic accidents may rise initially: Following the spring shift to daylight savings time, when one hour of sleep is lost, studies have found a measurable increase in the number of fatal accidents. Lost productivity is another short-term drawback, as sleep-disrupted workers adjust to the schedule change.

Finnish researchers have found that the transition to daylight savings time reduces both our sleep duration and efficiency. They monitored the rest-activity cycles of ten adults for ten days a year over two years. After the transition they noted that sleep time was shortened by 60 minutes and sleep efficiency was reduced by 10 percent on average.

But on a positive note, depression rates are set to fall. Researchers from Quebec, Canada say sleeping late increases REM sleep, and excessive REM sleep is linked to depression. They reviewed two studies on depression and sunrise time in cities, and found it was "significantly correlated" with depression rates — later sunrise (corresponding to earlier rising times) was associated with less depression.

A study in the Journal of Periodontology suggests that a chance to enjoy extra daylight can extend the life and health of our teeth and bones. That's because our bodies get vitamin D through sun exposure. Vitamin D, along with calcium, is essential for preventing bone and teeth disorders.

Other environmental factors related to mental health

I. Preterm birth is associated with increased risk for psychiatric hospitalization

A 2012 study (22660967) found: "Preterm birth was significantly associated with increased risk of psychiatric hospitalization in adulthood (defined as ≥16 years of age) in a monotonic manner across a range of psychiatric disorders." Monotonic means, in this case, the earlier preterm, the greater the risk of hospitalization.

II. Bipolar disorder is slightly associated with season of birth

A 1997 study(9428062) found: "More than 250 studies, covering 29 Northern and five Southern Hemisphere countries, have been published on the birth seasonality of individuals who develop schizophrenia and/or bipolar disorder. Despite methodological problems, the studies are remarkably consistent in showing a 5-8% winter-spring excess of births for both schizophrenia and mania/bipolar disorder."

A 2015 study (25862378) is titled: **Influence of light exposure during early life on the age of onset of bipolar disorder**

> "More hours of daylight at the birth location during early life was associated with an older age of onset, suggesting reduced vulnerability to the future circadian challenge of the springtime increase in solar insolation at the onset location. Addition of the

minimum of the average monthly hours of daylight during the first 3 months of life improved the base model, with a significant positive relationship to age of onset."

III. Light at night prior to adolescence may increase anxiety

A 2016 study (27592634) with mice is titled, **"Dim light at night prior to adolescence increases adult anxiety-like behaviors."**

Mice are nocturnal so care is needed in extending this result to humans. The authors suggest that a disruption of the circadian rhythm is involved. The significant result is that the expression of two clock genes CLOCK and Rev-ERB were altered by the dim light at night and anxiety and fear behavior resulted. These are the genes responsible for the resetting of the circadian clock by exposure to light in the morning.

If your child won't sleep in a dark room, be sure the light you provide is free of blue light so it won't disrupt the child's circadian rhythm.

Summary of Chapter 4

While inherited mutations of circadian genes play an important role in predisposing individuals to bipolar disorder, environmental factors may control the expression and frequency of bipolar episodes. Environmental factors that either control or disrupt the circadian rhythm appear to have a dramatic effect on those with bipolar disorder.

Conscious control of a regular lifestyle may compensate for a weak circadian clock. Exposing the eyes to bright light, rich in blue light, at about the same time each morning and avoiding blue light at night (by using special light bulbs or by wearing orange glasses), may help avoid bipolar episodes.

CHAPTER 5

Is Bipolar Disorder Progressive?

There are more than 300 scientific papers that suggest bipolar disorder is progressive, meaning that the disorder may get worse over time. Fortunately, not everyone with bipolar disorder will experience a progression of the disorder. It is important to recognize the fact that damage to the brain appears to occur during episodes of depression or mania. Thus, avoiding episodes of mania and depression becomes the goal of treatment.

Episode recurrence rate may increase with time

One of the early (1999) studies (10084757) found:

> "Survival analysis was used to calculate the rate of recurrence after successive episodes in a case register study including all hospital admissions with primary affective disorder in Denmark during 1971-1993. Totally, 20,350 first-admission patients were discharged with a diagnosis of affective disorder, depressive or manic/circular type. The rate of recurrence increased with the number of previous episodes in both unipolar and bipolar disorder. Initially, the two types of disorders followed markedly different courses, but later in the course of the illness the rate of recurrence was the same for the two disorders. The course of severe unipolar and bipolar disorder seems to be progressive in nature despite the effect of treatment."

A 2000 study (11166092) found:

> "We undertook a retrospective assessment of 426 inpatients affected by major depressive disorder (n=182) and bipolar disorder (n=244), with at least two episodes of illness alternating with complete recovery; subjects were affected for an average of 14.43+/-11.34 years and presented an average of 4.4+/-2.1 episodes. Random regression model analysis (http://www.uic.eu/hedeker/mix.html) was used to investigate the longitudinal time course of the illness. A progressive cycle-shortening was observed, whereby the more episodes a subject experienced, the shorter the interval was between episodes, up to a plateau frequency of one episode/year on average. Bipolar diagnosis was the strongest predictive factor toward high frequency of episodes; a manic onset among bipolars was associated with an even worse outcome. Gender, education level, family history, duration of the first interval, severity of the first episode, lifetime mean severity and lifetime mean treatment level were not associated with outcome in terms of episode frequency. Our results suggest that recurrent affective disorders recruited in a clinical setting have a marked deteriorating mean time course"

MRI studies show brain damage may occur during episodes

A 2003 MRI (brain imaging) study (21206844) found the size of the third ventricle (open area at center of brain) is significantly larger and increased in size, over time, in people with bipolar disorder.

Another MRI study (2005) (15777357) found:

> "Available findings suggest reduced grey matter in prefrontal brain regions such as anterior cingulate and subgenual prefrontal cortex, and abnormalities in amygdala size in adult and paediatric bipolar patients. White matter hyperintensities, which are

non-specific abnormalities, are also common in bipolar patients. Bipolar patients may lose more brain grey matter by ageing. There is also evidence for impaired myelination of the corpus callosum in bipolar disorder. Lithium may reverse or prevent grey matter prefrontal cortex abnormalities in bipolar patients by its neuroprotective effects."

A 2005 study (16318818) concluded:

"In all four studies, an effect of episodes was found in depressive (four studies) and bipolar (three studies) disorders. It is concluded that the average risk of recurrence increases with the number of episodes in depressive and in bipolar affective disorders."

A 2007 study (17617389) found:

"Patients with BPD showed a larger decline in hippocampal, fusiform, and cerebellar gray matter density over 4 years than control subjects. No significant changes in white matter density were found. Reductions in temporal lobe gray matter correlated with decline in intellectual function and with the number of intervening mood episodes over the follow-up period"

A 2009 study (19482934) found:

"Previous cross-sectional study of ventral prefrontal cortex (VPFC) implicated progressive volume abnormalities during adolescence in bipolar disorder (BD). In the present study, a within-subject, longitudinal design was implemented to examine brain volume changes during adolescence/young adulthood. We hypothesized that VPFC volume decreases over time would be greater in adolescents/young adults with BD than in healthy comparison adolescents/young adults. Eighteen adolescents/young adults (10 with BD I and 8 healthy comparison participants) underwent two high-resolution magnetic resonance imaging scans over approximately 2 years. Regional volume changes over time were measured. Adolescents/young adults with BD displayed significantly greater volume loss over time, compared to healthy comparison participants, in a region encompassing VPFC and rostral PFC and extending to rostral anterior cingulate cortex (p < .05). Additional areas where volume change differed between groups were observed. While data should be interpreted cautiously due to modest sample size, this study provides preliminary evidence to support the presence of accelerated loss in VPFC and rostral PFC volume in adolescents/young adults with BD."

Not all studies agree
A 2010 study (20433320) showed:

"Emerging neuroimaging data suggests that, in contrast to schizophrenia, where at the time of a first-episode of illness there is already discernible volume loss, in bipolar disorder, gross brain structure is relatively preserved, and it is only with recurrences that there is a sequential, but marked loss of brain volume. Recent evidence suggests that both pharmacotherapy and psychotherapy are more effective if instituted early in the course of bipolar disorder, and that with multiple episodes and disease progression there is a noticeable decline in treatment response." This argues for early intervention.

2011 study (21843279) used MRI to examine changes in grey matter volume (GMV).

"We observed increases in GMV in bipolar disorder subjects across several brain regions at baseline and over time, including portions of the prefrontal cortex as well as limbic and subcortical structures. Time-related changes differed to some degree between adolescent and adult bipolar disorder subjects. The interval between scans positively correlated with GMV increases in bipolar disorder subjects in portions of the prefrontal cortex, and both illness duration and number of depressive episodes were associated with increased GMV in subcortical and limbic structures. Our findings support suggestions that widely observed progressive neurofunctional changes in bipolar disorder patients may be related to structural brain abnormalities in anterior limbic structures. Abnormalities largely involve regions previously noted to be integral to emotional expression and regulation, and appear to vary by age."

A 2012 study (21943930) followed 128 BDI patients for 5.7 years with an average of 6.5 episodes per person. They found no evidence that the frequency of episodes increased over time. They reviewed 40 earlier studies and found only one third of them found shorter intervals of wellness between episodes. These were their patients so were receiving treatment. This is an encouraging trend.

Another 2012 study(23090632) states:

"In the present study, we review neuroanatomical evidence of the progression that occurs in many cases of BD, as well as cellular resilience mechanisms and peripheral biomarkers associated with distinct stages of this disorder. In summary, cellular resilience mechanisms seem to be less efficient at later stages of BD, especially mitochondrial and endoplasmic reticulum-related responses to stress. These insights may help in developing staging models of BD, with a special emphasis on the search for biomarkers associated with illness progression".

A 2013 study (23726659) compared cognitive ability in 24 BD type1 patients who were sixty years old or older with 20 BD type1 patients forty years old or younger. They found no evidence of a progressive decline.

2013 study (23449001) measured DNA oxidation in people with BD type I:

> "DNA levels of 8-OHdG, 5-HMec and 5-Mec were measured in 50 BD type I patients and 50 healthy controls. DNA 8-OHdG levels were higher in BD patients compared to healthy controls and found to be positively influenced by number of previous manic episodes. BD subjects had lower levels of 5-HMec compared to controls, whereas this measure was not influenced by the clinical features of BD. Number of manic episodes was correlated with higher levels of 8-OHdG, but not of 5-Mec or 5-HMec. Lower demethylation activity (5-HMec) but no difference in global 5-Mec levels was observed in BD. This finding suggests that oxidative damage to 8-OHdG might be a potential marker of disease progression, although further prospective cross-sectional studies to confirm neuroprogression in BD are warranted."

A 2015 study (26373602) examined the question of whether brain damage occurs as a result of manic episodes:

> "We followed patients with bipolar disorder type I for 6 years. Structural brain magnetic resonance imaging scans were performed at baseline and follow-up. We compared patients who had at least one manic episode between baseline and follow-up (Mania group, n = 13) with those who had no manic episodes (No-Mania group, n = 18). We used measures of cortical volume, thickness, and area to assess grey matter changes between baseline and follow-up. We found significantly decreased frontal cortical volume (dorsolateral prefrontal and inferior frontal cortex) in the Mania group, but no volume changes in the No-Mania group. Our results indicate that volume decrease in frontal brain regions can be attributed to the incidence of manic episodes."

This underscores the importance of avoiding or minimizing manic episodes.

A 2015 study (26645741) reported:

> "We used MRI to measure cortical volume, thickness and area in patients with BDI and BDII as well as in healthy controls. The large study cohort enabled us to adjust for important confounding factors. We included 81 patients with BDI, 59 with BDII and 85 controls in our analyses. Cortical volume, thickness and surface area abnormalities were present in frontal, temporal and medial occipital regions in patients with BD. Lithium and antiepileptic drug use had an effect on the observed differences in medial occipital regions. Patients with the subtypes BDI and BDII displayed common cortical abnormalities, such as lower volume, thickness and surface area than healthy controls in frontal brain regions but differed in temporal and medial prefrontal regions, where only those with BDI had abnormally low cortical volume and thickness."

This study does not address progression of the disorder but points out that BDII (no mania) appears to result in less brain damage.

A 2017 review paper (27858964) stated:

> "The objective of the present systematic literature review was to present evidence for associations between number of affective episodes and (i) the risk of recurrence of episodes, (ii) probability of recovery from episodes, (iii) severity of episodes, (iv) the threshold for developing episodes, and (v) progression of cognitive deficits in unipolar and bipolar disorders. Most of the five areas are superficially investigated and hampered by methodological challenges. Nevertheless, studies with the longest follow-up periods, using survival analysis methods, taking account of the

individual heterogeneity, all support a clinical progressive course of illness. Overall, increasing number of affective episodes seems to be associated with (i) increasing risk of recurrence, (ii) increasing duration of episodes, (iii) increasing symptomatic severity of episodes, (iv) decreasing threshold for developing episodes, and (v) increasing risk of developing dementia. Conclusion: Although the course of illness is heterogeneous, there is evidence for clinical progression of unipolar and bipolar disorders."

A 2017 study (27207915) concludes "Our findings showed that the serum of patients with bipolar disorder induced a decrease in neurite density and cell viability in neuronal cultures." The blood was from older patients with advanced stage of the disorder. The blood contained something that was damaging to neurons (brain cells). Blood from healthy people did not damage the brain cells.

A 2017 study (28628780) found:

"Using structural MRI data and BrainAGE quantification of acceleration or deceleration of in individual aging, we analysed data from 45 schizophrenia patients, 22 bipolar I disorder patients (mostly with previous psychotic symptoms / episodes), and 70 healthy controls. We found significantly higher BrainAGE scores in schizophrenia, but not bipolar disorder patients. Our findings indicate significantly accelerated brain structural aging in schizophrenia, but not in bipolar disorder."

Melatonin provides protection from brain damage

The numerous studies just cited suggest that brain damage may occur during bipolar episodes, but do not describe a detailed mechanism as to how this damage is caused. In my recent book, "Concussion" (available at www.lowbluelights.com or at Amazon), I quote many studies in which reactive oxygen and nitrogen species are shown to be responsible for damage to the brain. I also quote studies showing that melatonin is a powerful antioxidant that protects the brain from damage. These studies suggest that maximizing natural melatonin will help heal an injured brain.

A 2012 study (22694957) is titled, **"Genetic and functional abnormalities of the melatonin biosynthesis pathway in patients with bipolar disorder."** They found variants in the gene rs4446909 were associated with both bipolar disorder and low values of serotonin (required to make melatonin), but not with healthy controls.

A 2014 study (25012620) is titled **"Local melatonin regulates inflammation resolution: a common factor in neurodegenerative, psychiatric and systemic inflammatory disorders."** It describes how low values of melatonin are frequently found in psychiatric conditions and how some antipsychotic drugs boost serotonin production (precursor of melatonin) as a mechanism of their action.

A 2014 study (24959861) is titled **"The protective effect of melatonin against brain oxidative stress and hyperlocomotion in a rat model of mania induced by ouabain"**. They found melatonin not only protected the brain, but also reduced manic symptoms.

A 2014 study (24553808) describes the direct path from the pineal gland (where melatonin is produced) to the center of the brain, resulting in the concentration of melatonin in the cerebrospinal fluid being higher than that in the blood stream. This direct injection of melatonin into the brain is why maximizing natural melatonin is so significant.

These studies suggest that those with bipolar disorder may suffer from a less than normal supply of melatonin. This can contribute to bipolar symptoms and result in brain damage from reactive oxygen and nitrogen species. Therefore, it is important for individuals with bipolar disorder to maximize natural melatonin. Use of melatonin supplements (pills or liquid) should be considered during bipolar episodes.

Summary of Chapter 5
Not everyone with bipolar disorder will experience an increase in the frequency or severity of episodes. In addition, not all will experience a decline in cognitive ability or a measurable (by MRI) loss of brain function. However, the brain damage that does occur with some patients appears to occur during episodes of mania or depression. The goal, for many reasons, is to strive for stability and reduce brain injury. Individuals with bipolar disorder may benefit from the brain-healing effects of melatonin. In the next chapter, we will discuss treatments for bipolar disorder, including how to boost melatonin levels, as well as recommendations for pharmaceuticals and a healthy lifestyle.

CHAPTER 6

Treating Bipolar Disorder

Bipolar disorder (bd) can result from mutations in many different genes. This suggests that bd should not be regarded as a particular disorder but rather, as many different disorders, depending on which genes carry a mutation. One should not assume that the treatment that is beneficial for one case would work in another.

Lithium

The use of lithium to treat bipolar disorder began in the 1940's and is considered the "gold standard" treatment. It is used continuously by about a third of bd patients. We will examine the evidence concerning how it works and the numerous problems associated with its side effects. If one searches PubMed for "lithium bipolar disorder", one finds more than 7000 technical abstracts.

A 2017 study (28095742) examined core clock gene expression (there are 17 core clock genes) with and without lithium in bd patients who were lithium non-responders and lithium strong responders. After 2 days of lithium treatment, 8 of the responder's genes showed a change in expression while none of the non-responder's genes were affected. After 4 days just one gene (different from the 8) of the responders changed expression. Non-responder's genes showed no change. At 8 days only non- responder's genes showed a change in four genes only one of which (CRY1) had changed at 4 days in the responders. This suggests the bd of the responders involves one or more of the 8 genes mentioned. The bd of the non-responders involves one or more of the four different genes mentioned except for CRY1, which may or may not be related to either type of bd. It further suggests that lithium is effective because it cancels out the effect of the mutation in one or more of the eight genes mentioned above.

The rapidly increasing knowledge of the genetic basis of bipolar disorder holds promise for highly individualized treatment, similar to what is happening in cancer treatment.

A 2011 study (28117843) examined the protective effect of lithium in reducing damage to white matter in the brain following a first episode of mania. A second mood stabilizer quetiapine did not prevent damage. This neuro-protective role for lithium is in addition to its mood stabilizing effect.

A 2016 review paper (27003509) examined 95 studies of the impact of lithium (Li) treatment on mood disorders:

> "Li: acts directly on the molecular clocks; delays the phase of sleep-wakefulness rhythms and the peak elevation of diurnal cycle body temperature; reduces the amplitude and shortens the duration of activity rhythms and lengthens free-running rhythms. Chronic Li treatment stabilizes free-running activity rhythms, by improving day-to-day rhythmicity of the activity, with effects that appear to be dose related. Pharmacogenetics demonstrate several associations of Li's response with circadian genes (NR1D1, GSK3□, CRY1, ARNTL, TIM, and PER2). Finally, Li acts on the retinal-hypothalamic pineal pathway, influencing light sensitivity and melatonin secretion. Li is a highly investigated chronobiologic agent, and although its chronobiological effects are not completely understood, it seems highly likely that they constitute an inherent component of its therapeutic action in the treatment of mood disorders."

A 2017 study (28621334) is titled "**Telomere Length and Bipolar Disorder**". Telomeres are the tails at the end of a strand of DNA that tend to shorten each time a cell divides. Telomere length is a factor that can be inherited. It is currently being considered as a promising biomarker (indicator) of susceptibility to psychiatric disorders. They measured telomere length on 63 patients with BD, 74 first-degree relatives (49 relatives had no lifetime psychopathology and 25 had a non-BD mood disorder), and 80 unrelated healthy individuals. Participants also underwent magnetic resonance imaging to determine hippocampal volumes and cognitive assessment to evaluate episodic memory using the verbal paired associates test. Telomere length was shorter in psychiatrically well relatives ($p=0.007$) compared with unrelated healthy participants. (The smaller the p-value the more likely the result is real. 0.05 is considered marginal). Telomere length was also shorter in relatives (regardless of psychiatric status; $p<0.01$) and patients with BD not on lithium ($p=0.02$) compared with lithium-treated patients with BD. In the entire sample, telomere length was positively associated with left and right hippocampal volume and with delayed recall (shorter telomere correlated with smaller volume). This study provides evidence that shortened telomere length is associated with familial risk for BD. Lithium may have neuroprotective properties that require further investigation using prospective designs.

Another 2017 paper (28500272) with more than 30 authors from multiple universities purports to identify the molecular basis of bipolar disorder and identify the details of how lithium affects the disorder. A free copy of the full paper is available from the abstract. This increased knowledge may make it possible to exploit new ways to control the disorder.

Side Effects of Lithium
Common

- confusion, poor memory, or lack of awareness
- fainting

- fast or slow heartbeat
- frequent urination
- increased thirst
- irregular pulse
- stiffness of the arms or legs
- trouble breathing (especially during hard work or exercise)
- unusual tiredness or weakness
- weight gain

Rare

- blue color and pain in the fingers and toes
- coldness of the arms and legs
- dizziness
- eye pain
- headache
- noise in the ears
- vision problems

Long term

- kidney damage

Richard L. Hansler PhD

Use of repetitive tasks to prevent bipolar disease

The following article explores the possibility of retraining parts of the brain to reduce individual's susceptibility to bipolar disease

"Simple tasks can 'rewire' brains at risk of developing bipolar disorder"

Helen McArdle _Health Correspondent   Evening Times (Glasgow)

Simple tasks can "rewire" the brain in patients at a high genetic risk of developing bipolar disorder, according to research presented in Edinburgh.

The pilot study in New York offers hope of a low-cost early intervention which could prevent the onset of bipolar disease — also known as manic depression — potentially saving the health service money and allowing patients to avoid mood-stabilizing drugs known for their unpleasant side effects.

On average, one per cent of the population will require treatment for bipolar disorder but a person's risk of developing the disease is significantly higher if a parent or sibling already has it.

However, not all members of a family will fall ill and scientists want to understand what makes some people "resilient" despite their genetic predisposition.

Researchers in New York used a type of brain scan known as functional magnetic resonance imaging (MRI) to map activity in the brains of three groups: patients with bipolar disorder, their siblings who did not develop the illness, and unrelated healthy individuals.

They found that both the bipolar patients and their siblings had similar abnormalities in the areas of the brain involved in processing emotion, but that this appeared to change in siblings during the study.

Participants were asked to perform repetitive tasks on the computer for around two to three minutes every day, designed to tap into the parts of the brain compromised in bipolar disease – such the ability to regulate emotion, impulsivity, ambiguity and inhibitions.

Speaking at the Royal College of Psychiatrists International Congress in Edinburgh, Sophia Frangou, Professor of psychiatry at the Ichan Medical Institute, said: "This is an area of work I think you will see more and more. The pilot study gives patients simple task to do regularly at home.

"If they engage in these for about two minutes per day we do see a restructuring of the brain in a way that could be useful. It may actually be therapeutic and is actually cost effective."

"The tasks do not challenge them in the way that cognitive behavioural therapy [CBT] does, for example.

"That's not to dismiss CBT, but this is a very repetitive task. They have to train themselves to do it every day, but it involves very basic affective stimuli that have no significance to them.

"We know that if they do it for about three weeks there's a change, but we don't know how long that lasts. It will probably require booster sessions but we don't know how often these may be required. You have to think of it like going to the gym – you don't go to the gym for three weeks and expect the effects to last."

Artificial Intelligence Key to Treating Illness

UC and one of its graduates have teamed up to use artificial intelligence to analyze the fMRIs of bipolar patients to determine treatment.

Ann Thompson / WVXU

Complex computer software may be the key to correctly diagnosing and treating patients with various diseases.

Dr. Nick Ernest, a UC graduate who beat the Air Force in a simulated game of aerial combat with his artificial intelligence (AI) system, is now applying the concept to the human body.

In a proof of concept study, Ernest harnessed the power of his Psibernetix AI program to determine if bipolar patients could benefit from a certain medication. Using fMRIs of bipolar patients, the software looked at how each patient would react to lithium.

Fuzzy Logic appears to be very accurate

The computer software predicted with 100 percent accuracy how patients would respond. It also predicted the actual reduction in manic symptoms after the lithium treatment with 92 percent accuracy.

UC psychiatrist David Fleck partnered with Ernest and Dr. Kelly Cohen on the study. Fleck says without AI, coming up with a treatment plan is difficult. "Bipolar disorder is a very complex genetic disease. There are multiple genes and not only are there multiple genes, not all of which we understand and know how they work, there is interaction with the environment."

Ernest emphasizes the advanced software is more than a black box. It thinks in linguistic sentences. "So at the end of the day we can go in and ask the thing why did you make the prediction that you did? So it has high accuracy but also the benefit of explaining exactly why it makes the decision that it did."

More tests are needed to make sure the artificial intelligence continues to accurately predict medication for bipolar patients.

Artificial Intelligence could work for other diseases

Ernest says there's no reason this wouldn't work for other illnesses.

"It almost doesn't matter what the application is. This could have easily been whether this person responded well to a surgery or a different drug. With my company, we use this methodology with determining costs and markets, maintenance for machinery. Really any sort of predictive analytics or big learning type application could utilize this."

Ernest has started another study. It's to predict recovery rates for people who have had a concussion.

END OF QUOTATION.

Sleep Deprivation

The abstract of this 2014 paper (24345382) is printed here as a clear description of the power of combining chronotherapy with medication:

Rapid treatment response of suicidal symptoms to lithium, sleep deprivation, and light therapy (chronotherapeutics) in drug-resistant bipolar depression.

J Clin Psychiatry. 2014 Feb;75(2):133-40. doi: 10.4088/JCP.13m08455.

Benedetti F1, Riccaboni R, Locatelli C, Poletti S, Dallaspezia S, Colombo C.

Abstract

BACKGROUND:

One third of patients with bipolar disorder attempt suicide. Depression in bipolar disorder is associated with drug resistance. The efficacy of antidepressants on suicidality has been questioned. Total sleep deprivation and light therapy prompt a rapid and stable antidepressant response in bipolar disorder.

METHOD:

We studied 143 consecutively admitted inpatients (December 2006-August 2012) with a major depressive episode in the course of bipolar disorder (DSM-IV criteria). Among the 141 study completers, 23% had a positive history of attempted suicide and 83% had a positive history of drug resistance. During 1 week, patients were administered 3 consecutive total sleep deprivation cycles (each composed of a period of 36 hours awake followed by recovery sleep) combined with bright light therapy in the morning for 2 weeks. At admission, patients who had been taking lithium continued it, and those who had not been taking lithium started it. Severity of depression was rated according to the Hamilton Depression Rating Scale (HDRS) (primary outcome measure) and Beck Depression Inventory (BDI).

RESULTS:

Two patients switched polarity. Among the 141 who completed the treatment, 70% achieved a 50% reduction in HDRS score in 1 week, which persisted 1 month after in 55%. The amelioration involved an immediate and persistent decrease in suicide scores soon after the first total sleep deprivation cycle ($F_{3,411} = 42.78$, $P < .00001$). A positive history of suicide attempts was associated with worse early life stress and with worse suicide scores at baseline, but it did not influence response. Patients with current suicidal thinking or planning responded equally well ($F_{3,42} = 20.70$, $P < .000001$). Remarkably, however, non-responders achieved a benefit, with significantly decreased final scores also including suicidality ratings ($F_{3,120} = 6.55$, $P = .0004$). Self-ratings showed the same pattern of change. Previous history of drug resistance did not hamper response. During the following month, 78 of 99 responders continued to stay well and were discharged from the hospital on lithium therapy alone.

CONCLUSIONS:

The combination of total sleep deprivation, light therapy, and lithium is able to rapidly decrease depressive suicidality and prompt antidepressant response in drug-resistant major depression in the course of bipolar disorder.

Light Therapy

It is believed that bipolar disorder is associated with mutations in genes that are part of the circadian clock. Therefore, efforts to compensate for this deficit in the circadian clock by living a well regulated life style, may be of benefit across the spectrum of bd cases. Getting up and exposing the eyes to light (especially blue light) at about the same time every day should help. Showering, working, eating, exercising, relaxing. and blocking blue light in the evening, all at a consistent time, may help to avoid triggering an episode. The goal is to minimize episodes.

Light therapy in the early morning is considered standard treatment for Seasonal Affective Disorder (SAD), also called winter blues or winter depression. Its effectiveness with bipolar depression, when used alone, is not well established. In the previously mentioned study, we saw it used successfully when combined with other therapy. A 2012 study (22424890) compared light therapy to negative ion therapy (placebo) in patients with bipolar depression and found no difference between groups.

In healthy people, the ability of light (especially blue light) to reset the circadian clock in the early morning is well established. It may well be that the mutations in the various clock genes producing bipolar disorder involve this resetting (or failure to reset) by light in some bipolar disorder patients.

This 2015 paper (25839643) from the Harvard Review of Psychiatry titled "**The Psychiatry of Light**" represents the ultimate authority:

> "Bright light therapy and the broader realm of chronotherapy remain underappreciated and underutilized, despite their empirical support. Efficacy extends beyond seasonal affective disorder and includes nonseasonal depression and sleep disorders, with emerging evidence for a role in treating attention-deficit/hyperactivity disorder, delirium, and dementia."

Dark Therapy

A 1998 case study (9611672) of a man with rapid cycling bipolar disorder is described in the abstract as follows:

"BACKGROUND:

> The modern practice of using artificial light to extend waking activities into the nighttime hours might be expected to precipitate or exacerbate bipolar illness, because it has been shown that modifying the timing and duration of sleep can induce mania in susceptible individuals. With this possibility in mind, we treated a patient with rapidly cycling bipolar illness by creating an environment that was likely to increase and to stabilize the number of hours that he slept each night.

METHODS:

> We asked the patient to remain at bed rest in the dark for 14 hours each night (later this was gradually reduced to 10 hours).

Over a period of several years, his clinical state was assessed with twice-daily self-ratings, once-weekly observer ratings, and continuous wrist motor activity recordings. Times of sleeping and waking were recorded with sleep logs, polygraphic recordings, and computer-based event recordings.

RESULTS:

The patient cycled rapidly between depression and mania and experienced marked fluctuations in the timing and duration of sleep when he slept according to his usual routine, but his sleep and mood stabilized when he adhered to a regimen of long nightly periods of enforced bed rest in the dark.

CONCLUSIONS:

Fostering sleep and stabilizing its timing by scheduling regular nightly periods of enforced bed rest in the dark may help to prevent mania and rapid cycling in bipolar patients."

A 2005 study (15654938) is titled "Dark Therapy for Mania: A Pilot Study". The abstract states, in part:

"METHOD:

We exposed 16 bipolar inpatients affected by a manic episode to a regimen of 14 h of enforced darkness from 6 p.m. to 8 a.m. each night for three consecutive days [dark therapy (DT)]. Pattern of mood changes were recorded with the Young Mania Rating Scale (YMRS) and compared with a control group of 16 inpatients matched for age, sex, age at onset, number of previous illness episodes and duration of current episode, and were treated with therapy as usual (TAU).

RESULTS:

Adding DT to TAU resulted in a significantly faster decrease of YMRS scores when patients were treated within 2 weeks from the onset of the current manic episode. When duration of current episode was longer, DT had no effect. Follow-up confirmed that good responders needed a lower dose of antimanic drugs and were discharged earlier from the hospital.

CONCLUSIONS:

Chronobiological interventions and control of environmental stimuli can be a useful add-on for the treatment of acute mania in a hospital setting."

Blocking Blue Light

A 2005 study (15713707) is titled "Blocking low-wavelength light prevents nocturnal melatonin suppression with no adverse effect on performance during simulated shift work." This study showed that blocking blue light from entering the eye, made the body act as if in darkness, "virtual darkness".

In 2008, Dr. James Phelps proposed (17637562) that dark therapy becomes a practical treatment for bipolar mania by using blue blocking glasses to create virtual darkness. Patients can carry on normal evening activities while wearing the glasses rather than spending four hours in total darkness before going to bed.

The abstract of a 2014 study (25264124) by Dr. Henricksen of Norway is shown here in its entirety because of its dramatic impact:

Blocking blue light during mania - markedly increased regularity of sleep and rapid improvement of symptoms: a case report.

Bipolar Disord. 2014 Dec;16(8):894-8. doi: 10.1111/bdi.12265. Epub 2014 Sep 27.

Henriksen TE1, Skrede S, Fasmer OB, Hamre B, Grønli J, Lund A.

Author information

1

Department of Clinical Medicine, Section for Psychiatry, Faculty of Medicine and Dentistry, University of Bergen, Bergen, Norway; Division of Mental Health Care, Valen Hospital, Fonna Local Health Authority, Norway and MoodNet Research Group, Bergen, Norway; Division of Psychiatry, Haukeland University Hospital, Bergen, Norway.

Abstract

OBJECTIVE:

Available pharmacological treatment of mania is insufficient. Virtual darkness therapy (blue light-blocking treatment by means of orange-tinted glasses) is a promising new treatment option for mania. The basis for this might be the recently identified blue light-sensitive retinal photoreceptor, which is solely responsible for light stimulus to the circadian master clock. This is the first case report describing the clinical course of a closely monitored, hospitalized patient in a manic episode first receiving clear-lensed, and then blue light-blocking glasses.

METHODS:

A 58-year-old Caucasian man, with bipolar I disorder and three previous manic episodes, was hospitalized during a manic episode. In addition to pharmacological treatment, he was treated with clear-lensed glasses for seven days, then one day without glasses, followed by six days of blue light-blocking glasses. During the entire observational period, he wore an actigraph with internal light sensors.

RESULTS:

Manic symptoms were unaltered during the first seven days. The transition to the blue-blocking regime was followed by a rapid and sustained decline in manic symptoms accompanied by a reduction in total sleep, a reduction in motor activity during sleep intervals, and markedly increased regularity of sleep intervals. The patient's total length of hospital stay was 20 days shorter than the average time during his previous manic episodes.

CONCLUSIONS:

The unusually rapid decline in symptoms, accompanied by uniform sleep parameter changes toward markedly increased regularity, suggest that blue-blockers might be targeting a central mechanism in the pathophysiology of mania that needs to be explored both in clinical research and in basic science.

In 2016 Dr. Henricksen published a study (27226262) in which 23 patients who were hospitalized for bipolar mania, were assigned (at random) either clear or orange glasses (from www.lowbluelights.com). They were required to wear the glasses or to be in darkness for a total of 14 hours each night. The results are described in this article from NEWSWEEK.

NEWSWEEK

08/19/16

Light from the sun helps to synchronize the internal clock, while artificial light from phones and TVs can mess up the natural biological rhythm. Glasses the block blue light might be able to help treat mental illnesses such as bipolar disorder.

If you have bipolar disorder, depression or trouble sleeping, it may help to wear amber-tinted glasses at night, new research suggests. These orange shades block blue light, which the body uses to adjust the biological clock to control sleeping and many other functions.

Blue light is a major component of sunlight, and exposure to it in the morning signals that it's time to wake up and also helps reset the body's clock, which is why morning sun is so important for adjusting to jet lag. Likewise, darkness following sundown serves as a cue to sleep. This worked well for our ancestors whose primary source of light was the sun. But many modern-day electronic devices like phones, computers and televisions also emit blue light, and being exposed to these after dusk can confuse the body, interrupting sleep. This, in turn, can worsen and increase the risk of developing various mental illnesses.

Scientists have proposed that limiting exposure to blue light given off by electronics at night could help people sleep and help reset dysfunctional biological clocks, both of which are involved in disorders like manic depression.

In a small Norwegian study of 23 people hospitalized for bipolar disorder, scientists assigned 12 to wear "blue-blocking" amber glasses for one week, and 11 not to. Meanwhile, no changes were made to the patient's medications.

The paper found an enormous difference between the two groups. Those wearing the amber-tinted glasses for only one week scored on average 14 points lower on a test used to measure mania known as the Young Mania Rating Scale. That's more than twice what doctors consider to be a "clinically significant difference" and is a "remarkably high effect size," according to a commentary accompanying the study, both of which were published in the journal *Bipolar Disorders*. Improvements were noticeable after only three nights of wearing the sunglasses.

"I was surprised by the magnitude of changes and the rapid onset of improvement," says study first author Tone Henriksen, a researcher with the University of Bergen and Valen Hospital in Norway. Even drug treatments aren't typically known to lead to such quick and significant turnarounds, she adds. These are "knock-your-socks off results," says Dr. James Phelps, a researcher and psychiatrist with Samaritan Health Services in Corvallis, Oregon, who wasn't involved in the study. It's incredibly important to find new treatments as 20 percent of people with bipolar disorder commit suicide, the highest rate for any mental illness, he adds.

The paper builds on a growing body of research showing how important light is for controlling not only circadian rhythms but mood and many other aspects of physical and mental health. In the last couple decades, scientists discovered an entirely new type of receptor in the eye called intrinsically photo-responsive retinal ganglion cells.

These receptors detect only blue light and communicate with the hypothalamus, where the biological clock lives, explains Phelps. There are also connections with areas of the brain controlling the limbic system, involved in mood and anxiety disorders. Though research on amber-tinted lenses has been limited, it has been shown that by blocking blue light, they trick the brain into thinking that it is dark. This allows the brain's pineal gland to produce melatonin, an important hormone that helps promote sleep, Phelps explains.

It seems that several mental disorders are exacerbated by too much light, or an irregular cycle of light and dark, and this includes bipolar disorder.

In a 2009 study in *Chronobiology International*, Phelps and a colleague found that 50 percent of 20 bipolar patients experiencing insomnia had significant improvements in sleep after wearing blue-blocking glasses. The majority of those who responded showed not just small but dramatic improvements.

Other studies have shown that exposing bipolar patients to actual darkness during the nighttime can have similar results; one 2005 paper found that putting 16 bipolar patients in darkened rooms for 14 hours per day greatly improved their manic symptoms. But actual darkness is much more difficult to obtain, and more disruptive to life.

Studies have also shown that light can act as an antidepressant. One study in *JAMA Psychiatry* in January found that subjecting patients to bright light therapy was as effective at improving (unipolar) depression as the antidepressant fluoxetine, but with fewer side effects. And exposure to light can also help prevent the depressive phase of bipolar disorder, says Francesco Benedetti, a psychiatrist at San Raffaele Hospital in Milan uninvolved in the present study.

There is still much to be learned about dark and light therapy, but some psychiatrists are ready to recommend these techniques and blue-blocking glasses. "When you have a low-risk, almost no-cost treatment with high efficacy, it's time to just use it," Phelps says.

He adds that some of his colleagues would disagree with him, and he notes that it will be difficult to study the effect of the glasses once they are widely used. But people will find out about the glasses anyway via the internet, so "we might as well tell them what we know," he adds.

Light- and dark therapy, blue-blocking glasses, and interventions that shift around sleep and wake time can have huge impacts on bipolar disorder and depression, and Benedetti says that it's time to start using so-called "chronotherapeutics" more widely.

"It's time that these techniques enter the common, everyday clinical practice everywhere, as they do in several hospitals, mainly in Europe," Benedetti says.

End of NEWSWEEK article.

Social Rhythm Therapy

In a 2015 study (26614534) titled **"Social rhythm disrupting events increase the risk of recurrence among individuals with bipolar disorder"** they provide the evidence supporting this claim. This is part of the evidence that maintaining a strong, steady circadian rhythm, free of disruption by exposure to blue light at night, will help avoid episodes.

A second 2015 study (25346391) of 100 patients found that "Interpersonal and social rhythm therapy used as an adjunct to pharmacotherapy appeared to be effective in reducing depressive and manic symptoms and improving social functioning in adolescents and young adults with bipolar disorder."

Since it is now fairly well accepted that bipolar disorder involves the genes of the circadian clock, it should be no surprise that doing as much as possible to lead a stable life-style will reduce the burden of recurrent episodes of depression or mania. On the other hand, when stuck in a long period of depression, the radical nature of sleep deprivation therapy should not cause fear of trying it.

Summary of Chapter 6

There is no cure for bipolar disorder but treatment can greatly reduce the negative effects of the disorder. Many people with bipolar disorder lead virtually normal lives. Since episodes of both depression and mania can result in brain damage, it is important to strive for stability to avoid episodes and to minimize the intensity and duration of episodes.

Lithium and other drugs have proven very helpful in obtaining stability. Developing a well-established schedule for getting up, exposing the eyes to light, showering, eating breakfast, working, having lunch, working, and so forth, will also help to avoid episodes. Careful planning will help minimize stress of all kinds. In addition, maximizing natural melatonin by controlling exposure to blue light in the hours before bedtime will improve health for many reasons, including protecting the brain from damage, especially during episodes.

Given the broad spectrum of bipolar disorder, treatment must be personalized to the individual. This treatment may include drugs such as lithium, but should also incorporate a regulated healthy lifestyle and other potential treatments such as repetitive task training, light therapy, darkness therapy, blocking blue light, sleep deprivation therapy, and social rhythm therapy.

CHAPTER 7

The Bottom Line

What can the reader conclude from all of this? If you have been given the diagnosis of bipolar disorder, you, no doubt, asked "Why me?" We saw in Chapter 4 that bipolar disorder is clearly an inherited disorder in which the rules for how it is inherited are not yet clearly understood. Since mutations in one or more of a group of genes are involved, it is not just one disorder, but rather a spectrum of disorders. As our ability to measure an individual's genome improves (very likely in your lifetime), which mutation(s) you inherited will become known and your treatment tailored to your specific needs. In the meantime, many people with bipolar disorder live very normal lives and achieve great things as a result of finding a medication that helps them stabilize their mood.

There is a great deal of evidence that bipolar disorder is associated with defects in the circadian clock as a result of mutations in one or more of the genes that make up the circadian clock. This master clock in the SCN is primarily controlled by blue light striking the ipRGC in the retina first thing in the morning. The circadian clocks in the individual cells throughout the body can respond not only to the arrival of melatonin, sent out under control of the master clock, but to other time signals, resulting from when we eat, when we exercise, when we work, when we relax, etc.

If you have bipolar disorder, this information about resetting your circadian clock provides a way for you to take over some aspects of your life that your genes are not doing properly. This is a powerful idea. By regulating your lifestyle, you have the ability to manage part of the automatic control system that isn't working properly. With strategic planning and help from those around you, you can organize your daily life into a regular routine. Morning exposure of your eyes to light at about the same time every day is probably the most significant step toward a regular life style.

Poor sleep is not only a hallmark of bipolar disorder but of many mood disorders. In many cases, this can be attributed to a poorly-functioning internal clock. That is, it fails to provide melatonin flow 12 hours after the resetting of the clock in the morning. This may be a failure of the circadian clock itself. It may be because the eyes are exposed to light at the time when melatonin should start flowing. This type of disruption of the circadian cycle can be avoided by shielding the eyes with glasses that block the blue rays that cause melatonin suppression.

The use of these blue-light blocking glasses (also known as orange or amber glasses) is an easy way to control your circadian rhythm and improve your sleep. These orange glasses should be worn for a few hours before bedtime and at about the same time every evening. Putting on the glasses about three hours before a regular bedtime will avoid disrupting your circadian rhythm. You will be returning to the situation that existed when humans evolved hundreds of thousands of years ago. By blocking the blue rays, wearing the glasses will make your body react as if in darkness.

Since 2005, thousands of healthy people have purchased orange glasses at www.lowbluelights.com with a guarantee of money back if they do not improve their sleep. They help more than 90% of those who try them. We believe many of our customers are people with bipolar disorder for whom their doctors have suggested our glasses. Some have told us that use of the glasses helps to stabilize their mood in addition to improving their sleep. The powerful effect of these glasses on bipolar disorder was established by the experiment in Norway, where they helped patients with mania recover quickly while clear glasses provided no effect. (See Chapter 6)

The orange (amber) glasses may be useful to those with bipolar disorder

for two reasons. Avoiding melatonin suppression will enhance sleep, the most common symptom of mood disorders. A second reason may be to avoid brain stimulation caused by exposure of the eyes to blue light. Nerves from special cells in the retina have connections to the circadian clock as well as to centers in the brain that control alertness. Stimulating these nerves in the retina with blue light may bring on mania or hypomania. The orange glasses may help avoid this stimulation. Many of our customers say our orange glasses help calm them and help if they have a headache.

Maximizing natural melatonin is good for several reasons. Improving sleep is first. Reducing brain damage by avoiding manic episodes is second. A third reason to maximize the time when melatonin is produced is to avoid damage to the brain when bipolar episodes do occur. The pineal gland sends melatonin directly into the center of the brain. Because the brain is extremely active during mania, it is producing lots of reactive oxygen species (free radicals) that kill brain cells if not neutralized by antioxidants like melatonin. Eating lots of colorful fruits, nuts, and vegetables will also help provide antioxidants during the day when the pineal gland is not making melatonin.

The following article provides a good summary of how individuals with bipolar disorder can maintain control over their well-being, leading healthy and rewarding lives.

"Will I Ever Get Better?"
By Jeremy Schwartz LCSW

> While there's no "cure" for bipolar, that doesn't mean it's something you'll have to battle forever.

The Bottom Line

People with bipolar disorder are often misdiagnosed, and many go through multiple visits to psychiatrists and therapists and try several medications before receiving an accurate diagnosis and effective treatment. It's hard to get an accurate bipolar diagnosis because of the condition's very nature: People go through manic, hypomanic and depressive episodes at different times, but health care providers only see one of those episodes at a time.

Of course, it's important to give your health care provider as full and accurate a history as possible, but this can be difficult to do when you're going through a difficult time.

While there's no "cure" for bipolar, that doesn't mean it's something you'll have to battle forever. With the right treatment and self-care, you can live a healthy and fulfilling life.

Living well with bipolar is difficult, and people often face serious impairment in functioning. However, people can and do get better over time. One recently published study shows that self-management of bipolar symptoms plays a strong role in personal recovery. Another study concluded that empowering people to manage their mood and view mood changes as normal may facilitate recovery. According to the results, decreased negative beliefs about the illness are significantly correlated with improved recovery outcomes. Self-esteem and hopefulness are important to achieving recovery.

So, when your mood changes, don't despair. View it as something to take care of, use your self-management tools and work with your health care provider.

Bipolar disorder is believed to have a genetic component, but don't take that to mean there's nothing you can do. Increasing attention to the field of epigenetics – environmental factors that switch genes on and off – has shown that we have quite a bit of power in how our genes are expressed. Further, research into neuroplasticity shows that the brain can and does change over time. You aren't limited to your genes, your childhood experiences, nor to a diagnosis.

But don't stop treatment just yet. Recovery can be a long process, and stopping treatment too soon could set you back. Talk to your treatment team before making any changes. It's common for mood disorders to follow a cyclical pattern. You may be feeling better right now, but that doesn't mean you're cured.

Have you been diagnosed with bipolar disorder? Here are five key things you should know:

1. A diagnosis doesn't sentence you to a lifetime of suffering. It can actually be empowering.

Learning that you have bipolar disorder gives you valuable information about the difficulties you've been having and what they mean. There is effective treatment for bipolar disorder, plus lifestyle changes you can make to put yourself on the road to recovery. Through a combination of self-management and quality treatment, many people live well with bipolar disorder.

2. Medication can help, but it isn't a cure.

Self-care such as exercise, good nutrition and consistent sleep is also important. Tracking your mood and your self-care behaviors consistently will help you notice the earliest signs of relapse. Take these early signs seriously, and stay in contact with your health care providers so you can address them right away.

Work and meaningful activities can play a role, too. Anything you can do to build up your resilience will make you less vulnerable to negative emotional states.

3. Therapy and medication can work hand in hand.

For some people, a mood stabilizer such as lithium can offer a complete remission of symptoms. Bipolar often responds very well to medication, and stopping medication does come with a significant risk of relapse. Treatments such as dialectical behavior therapy and cognitive behavioral therapy are also promising. While medication helps stabilize your mood, therapy can help you develop new ways of thinking and being to create lasting change.

4. You'll need multiple sources of support.

Make sure to involve family members and friends, to the extent that they can be supportive and helpful. Let people know what you're going through and how they can help. You may also need to assert boundaries and set limits when people do things that aren't helpful. This can be uncomfortable at first, but there's nothing to feel guilty about when you set limits and assert your needs.

Peer support groups can also be a great resource. Organizations such as the National Alliance on Mental Illness and the Depression and Bipolar Support Alliance have local chapters and may offer free groups in your area. Participation in peer support groups can even reduce the need for hospitalization and other treatments.

5. Recovery is possible.

Recovery doesn't necessarily mean being symptom-free forever. But it can mean being able to live your life and achieve personally meaningful goals without bipolar having to be an insurmountable obstacle. Recovery is something you can define for yourself, based on what you care about.

END OF ARTICLE

Action

Knowledge has little value if it does not result in action. Learning all you can about bipolar disorder will help you to best manage your condition, with the support of medical professionals, family and friends.

Knowing that bipolar disorder is of genetic origin and that knowledge of genetics is expanding rapidly is very encouraging. Learning all you can about your genome should help your doctor provide the best treatment. In addition, you may wish to seek genetic counseling before making major life decisions.

Finally, joining support groups may be helpful not only to you but to others in the group. BP Magazine and newsletter are also good sources of new information regarding bipolar disorder.

Author's note

As the author, I wish you the very best. I hope that you have found this book to be a useful resource in gaining a better understanding of bipolar disorder, as well as providing practical suggestions for treatment.

I welcome your comments about the book at rhansler@jcu.edu or call me at 216 929 0227.

Richard L. Hansler

www.ingramcontent.com/pod-product-compliance
Lightning Source LLC
Chambersburg PA
CBHW070306230526
45470CB00002B/742